HEALING W

In the same series

Handbook Of Herbs

Uniform with this book

HEALING

WITHOUT HARM

(Pathways to Alternative Medicine)

by

E. G. BARTLETT

PAPERFRONTS
**ELLIOT RIGHT WAY BOOKS,
KINGSWOOD, SURREY, U.K.**

Made and Printed in Great Britain by Hunt Barnard Ltd, Aylesbury, Bucks.

CONTENTS

INTRODUCTION

Orthodox medicine relies heavily on drugs and surgery. Great successes are claimed for drugs, particularly in the fields of bacterial and parasitic infections; pneumonia and tuberculosis are no longer killer diseases; syphilis is curable. Drugs can relieve pain. Used as anaesthetics they make necessary surgical operations possible. They can prevent disease, as when someone going into a malarial area protects himself with quinine tablets before he sets out. We should never minimize the value of drugs in medicine. Diabetic patients would not be alive without their daily dose of insulin.

Certainly drugs do good, but there is another side. How much of the good attributed to them should rightly be attributed to improved hygiene and living conditions? How much of what we believe is due to companies with vested interests promoting drug therapies?

Drugs also do harm. They can harm the patient in various ways. There are side effects, for example drowsiness from pheno-barbitone, vomiting from digoxin or morphine, male sexual difficulties from drugs used to relieve high blood pressure. There are secondary effects, for example thrush when antibiotics eliminate natural bacterial flora in the bowel. There are toxic effects, not only from overdose, but from ordinary doses given to a patient with an underlying condition. There are adverse reactions between different drugs. The dramatic and disastrous effects of putting drugs on the market before they have been sufficiently tested was highlighted by the thalidomide case. The chemotherapy and the radium treatments used in cancer cases destroy healthy tissue as well as the cancerous growth they are seeking to eliminate, and often the patient suffers from vomiting and loss of appetite. Readers who wish to know more of the adverse effects of drug therapy are referred to Melville and

Johnson's book "Cured to Death" (Secker and Warburg 1982).

As well as the harm they do to man, drugs harm the thousands of laboratory animals on whom they must be tested before they can be released onto the market. In their book "The Medicine You Take" by Drs. D. R. Laurence and J. W. Black (Croom Helm 1978), the authors say "It is hard to doubt that, especially in toxicity testing, a lot of suffering is caused to conscious animals". The authors of this book are not against the tests; they believe them to be necessary. Their admission is therefore the more damning in the eyes of those who believe that they have no right to purchase their own health and happiness at the expense of the well-being of any other of God's creatures.

A moral dilemma clearly exists. Not only are laboratory animals used to test drugs; they are used to develop new skills and to demonstrate old skills to students. The number and the nature of these uses is rightly a matter for public concern. The cruelty involved is sometimes horrific.

Surgery deliberately and sometimes drastically harms the body, to achieve a good end, and it can go wrong. Any treatment that offers the slightest hope of avoiding surgery is therefore worth investigation.

This book is intended for all who seek healing without harm. They may reject our right to use animals for our own ends. They may refuse to accept that any treatment that harms their own body can ultimately do good. They may feel that there is something wrong with conventional medicine. They may have heard of other forms of healing from friends who have benefited. They may be turning elsewhere in despair because past treatment has not helped their case. Whatever their reason, it is worth their while to consider the claims of alternative medicine.

Much of what is called "alternative medicine" is in fact much earlier in origin and use than orthodox medicine, and it adopts a more natural approach to healing. Orthodox medicine treats people when they are ill, and preventive measures take a secondary place. Alternative medicine will treat people when they are well and seeks to prevent them becoming ill.

There are other differences between the two forms. Orthodox medicine mainly attacks the symptoms of the particular malady of which the patient is complaining. The alternative forms treat the whole man, seeking to relate his present condition to his whole life-style, which may need to be changed as part of the cure or to prevent a recurrence of the illness. This approach is of course also taught to orthodox medical students in their early training but it is soon lost when they go into general practice. Alternative medicine rejects synthetic drugs in the main, seeking to use natural remedies and to help the body to heal itself. The methods are gentler in approach to the patient and less violent in their action on his body.

Critics of these alternative forms point out that many of them are without scientific foundation. The meridians of Ch'i used in acupuncture for example, cannot be identified in anatomy. Nor can some of these alternative forms be subjected to the clinical tests that doctors impose on more orthodox treatments. Doctors will often use a placebo in their tests for example. This consists of giving one set of patients a drug whilst giving to another a substance that appears identical but which has no curative properties whatever. The results can then be compared. But such therapies as chiropractic, osteopathy or faith healing could never be tested in a similar way, because it is impossible to give fake adjustments to the spine or fake faith healing.

In this book, we shall look at the forms of alternative medicine that are generally available. Some, such as acupuncture, homoeopathy, herbalism, and naturopathy are well known and treat all kinds of illness. Others, such as aroma therapy are aids to healing rather than complete healing systems in themselves. Many practitioners of these alternative therapies do not like the use of the word "alternative", because it suggests a choice between one or the other. Some will easily combine with orthodox medical treatment, and certainly many of the alternative therapies will combine with each other.

This is in no sense a "Treat Yourself" book. Though you might use some of the methods (The Bach Flower Remedies for example), it might be positively dangerous to attempt to use some of the other techniques on yourself. The book is intended to be a guide to what is available for different purposes and to those bodies who can put you in touch with qualified practitioners. No attempt has been made to judge or assess the value of the therapies. In some cases the only possible way of judging would be to try them for yourself. The aim here is simply to present the history, philosophy, methods and claims of each system in turn, so that the reader can choose those he thinks worthy of further investigation.

Of these therapies, only homoeopathy is available on the National Health Service. Other treatments can be expensive, since they come within the private sector. It is therefore worth enquiring the fee before you start a course of treatment.

An advantage of going to an alternative therapist, however, is that he is likely to have more time to delve into the underlying causes of your complaint than a busy N.H.S. practitioner with a full surgery and a round of house calls waiting. The average time allowed per patient by a busy doctor is ten minutes; the minimum time with an alternative practitioner will be fifteen minutes and may well be up to a couple of hours.

Orthodox medicine tends to be severely mechanistic in its concepts, carrying over the materialistic thought of the last century. Even psychosomatic illness took some time to be recognised, and the term was being used scornfully as late as the 1950's. The relation of the spiritual element to total health is even less likely to interest doctors who have been taught that illness has physical causes and physical cures. Many of the alternative therapies bring the spiritual element to the fore, identifying healing as an activity of a benevolent life-force in the Universe, by whatever name it may be called, and seeking harmony with the teachings of the great world religions.

The approach of all the therapies in this book is holistic and gentle. Administered by properly qualified practitioners, none of them should cause harm. None of them involves experiments on animals. If treatment you have received in the past has not helped you, or if, on moral or ethical grounds, you seek healing without harm, it is worth reading further.

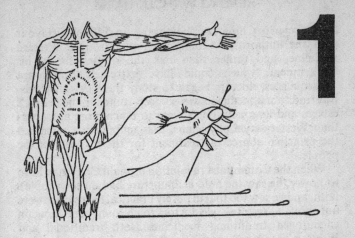

ACUPUNCTURE AND ACUPRESSURE

Acupuncture is one of the oldest forms of treatment. It is Chinese in origin, and dates back to at least 2697 B.C. when Huang Ti, the Father of Acupuncture, succeeded Shen Nung as Emperor. Huan Ti, with his doctor Ch'i Po, worked out the principles of anatomy and health on which the theory and practice of acupuncture is based. They were written down in a book called "Nei Ching", which has been translated as "The Yellow Emperor's Classic of Internal Medicine". The book is divided into two parts, the first dealing with the principles of medicine in relation to the Universe, the second with the actual practice of Acupuncture.

In 1822, a Court Decree struck acupuncture from the curriculum of the Imperial Medical College and it fell into disrepute and came to be practised by charlatans, though genuine practitioners still abounded, passing on their knowledge outside the medical colleges. During Chiang Kai

Shek's reign in China, acupuncture again suffered disfavour with the authorities. Chiang tried to introduce Western medicine, and rather than risk the displeasure of his Government, which could have extremely unpleasant consequences, doctors began to study these new methods. But traditional medicine was so deep-rooted in the people's esteem and its practitioners were so much more numerous than Western-style physicians, that acupuncture remained the principal source of treatment for the majority of the people.

When the Communist revolution brought Chairman Mao to power, he saw the hold acupuncture had on the people's faith, and he saw too that in purely practical terms there were not enough Western-style doctors to go round, and he again encouraged traditional medicine. Both traditional and Western medicine flourish in China today, and patients visiting a clinic will be given the choice as to which treatment they prefer.

Acupuncture is a holistic system of healing, in that it treats the whole man, not just his present condition. It is a system in tune with the Universe, and to understand it, we must understand something of Chinese philosophy.

The Chinese believe that there exists an invisible and indefinable life-force, to which they give the name "Ch'i". It is the motivating force behind the Universe, and has two forms of expression, Yin and Yang. All matter, including the human body and every part of it, is made up of Yin and Yang. Yin is the negative, yielding, feminine side of things; Yang is the positive, dominating, masculine.

Ch'i, the life-force, comes into the body at birth and leaves it at death. It flows around a system of meridians that extend through the torso and the limbs. These meridians are neither blood vessels nor nerves nor anything physical, and for this reason their very existence has been scoffed at by Western scientists. But the fact that neither the meridians nor Yin and Yang nor even Ch'i itself can be proved to exist is irrelevant, when the system of healing based on these concepts has worked for over 6000 years and still works today. Whatever names we give to these phenomena and however much they defy pinning down by laboratory tests, they are concepts that produce supremely practical results in terms of healing.

The flow of Ch'i in a man's body is not constant. It varies with the seasons, with the time of day, and even with the weather. Yin and Yang forever fluctuate, and for health they need not be equal in any part of the body; they need only be in the right balance. Illness, according to this philosophy, results from an imbalance of Yin and Yang, and is cured by restoring the balance, by use of the acupuncturist's needles.

Chinese philosophy teaches that Yin and Yang produce the five elements: wood, fire, earth, metal and water. Acupuncture theory links these five elements with the liver, the heart, the spleen, the lungs and the kidneys respectively. These are called solid organs; they have Yin characteristics, and their functions are internal.

Each of these solid organs has a corresponding hollow organ: the gall-bladder, the small intestine, the stomach, the large intestine, and the bladder. These are Yang in character.

According to the theory of acupuncture, there are two more organs in the body, neither of them known to Western medicine. These are "The Triple Warmer", a Yang organ, which has no definite form, but is simply a regulator of the flow of fluids between the other organs, and "The Gate of Life", a Yang organ said to be situated between the kidneys and to be the regulator of sex and circulation.

The acupuncturist sees man as fitting into the rhythms of the Universe, such as the seasonal rhythms, for example. Spring is a time of new beginning. New shoots come forth in the earth; they develop in Summer; they fruit in the Autumn; they die away in Winter. Spring is linked with wood and with the liver; Summer with fire and the heart; early Autumn with earth and the spleen; late Autumn with metal and the lungs; Winter with water and the kidneys. Just as there is an interaction between the seasons, one developing into the other, so there is interaction between the five elements and between the five organs of the body. As water destroys fire, so the kidneys can have a bad effect on the heart. As wood nourishes a fire, so the liver can have a good effect on the heart. This is simplifying the case of course, but it illustrates the kind of interaction the acupuncturist will consider when dealing with his patients.

Before going further, however, we should look at the kind of training an acupuncturist would receive. The Imperial Institute of Physicians, established in China in the Tang Dynasty during the 7th Century A.D. was the first medical school in the world. Through it, the State regulated medical practice. Untrained doctors were prohibited from practising. To qualify in this College, students had to take a two-day examination. The first day was devoted to an oral examination on the text of "Nei Ching" and on anatomy in general. A single mistake in this part of the examination could result in failure, but if the student passed this first ordeal, he went on to practical tests on the following day. For these practical tests, a life-sized wooden doll was used. It was so constructed that it was hollow and could be filled with water, and at each of the acupuncture points a small hole was bored. There were 365 of these points in those early dolls, corresponding to the days of the year. When prepared for use, the doll was coated with wax and filled with water. The wax hid the holes from the student and also kept the water from flowing out until the student inserted his needles. If he could insert them correctly, water would flow; if he could not find the exact spot, no water came out, and he would fail his examination.

The student taking this practical test would be given various cases to consider. He would be told the sex and the age of a patient, where he had been born, whether married or single, the season of the year and the time of day the consultation was taking place, since all these factors would have to be taken into account when deciding the treatment. The student would then say what he thought was wrong with the patient, and name the point or points where the insertion of needles would be beneficial. Then would come the dramatic moment when he was called upon to insert the needle into the doll. Success or failure was immediately apparent.

These dolls are still used in the training of an acupuncturist, though they are often made of metal or other materials now. Students also train by inserting the needles in themselves. Today, in China, there is a six year training course, though in earlier times, practitioners would sometimes learn from the village doctor as apprentices, rather than go to college themselves. The present day student has to be able to locate all these acupuncture points exactly, just as he did in the old days, and although there are more of them today, the original ones have not changed at all.

The acupuncture points all lie along the meridians of Ch'i. Just as the organs are divided into Yin and Yang organs, so the meridians are also divided. The sex meridian is Yin; it runs from the tip of the middle finger to the chest. The liver meridian is Yin; it runs from the end of the big toe up the leg into the trunk. The Triple Warmer meridian is Yang; it starts at the end of the third finger, runs up the arm and neck to the eye. The gall bladder meridian is Yang; it runs from the head down the body to the big toe. The lung meridian is Yin; it runs from the second rib up the shoulder and down the arm to the thumb. The spleen meridian is Yin; it runs from the big toe up the leg to the armpit. The small intestine meridian is Yang; it runs from the end of the little finger, and up the arm, across the back, up the neck to the ear. The bladder meridian is Yang; it runs from the nose, up over the top of the head, down the back of the body and leg to the last joint of the big toe. The large intestine meridian is Yang; it runs from the end of the index finger, up the arm to the face, and the corner of the mouth. The stomach meridian is Yang; it runs from the side of the head, down the body and leg to the second toe. The heart meridian is Yin; it runs from the top of the armpit down to the end of the little finger. The kidney meridian is Yin; it runs from the sole of the foot, up the leg, to the chest.

Ancient charts marked all these meridians and points along them on the same diagram, which makes them extremely difficult to follow. Modern charts split them up, with a separate meridian on a separate diagram. There are ancient sculptures too which give these meridians and points. Of course, the meridians mentioned are only the main ones. There are subsidiary meridians, and modern acupuncturists recognise fifty-nine of them and about a thousand points.

Because symptoms are linked with specific meridians, it has been possible to publish a list of acupuncture points to be used in treating various illnesses, and improperly trained practitioners might rely too much on these. The really skilled practitioner will use them only as very general guidelines, since there is so much more to be considered in treating a patient. The time of day, the season, the weather, all determine whether Yin or Yang is prevalent in nature. Whichever is most prevalent in the natural world will be the one most easily stimulated in the patient, since a human body at its healthiest is in tune with nature. Having decided where the imbalance lies, the practitioner must consider whether to rectify it by increasing Yang or decreasing Yin.

There are four laws to be considered. They are:

1. The Mother-Son Law. Ch'i is considered to flow through the body beginning in the lung meridian, and then passing on through the meridians of the large intestine, the stomach, the spleen, the heart, the small intestine, the bladder, the kidneys, the sex, the Triple Warmer, the gall bladder, and the liver meridians in that order. A meridian which precedes another in this list is said to be the "mother" of the one that follows; and the one that follows is of course the "son". The stomach meridian is thus the mother of the spleen meridian, and to increase activity in the spleen meridian, the acupuncturist can stimulate the stomach meridian with his needles. Note, it is the meridians we are considering, not the organs after which they are named.

2. The Husband-Wife Law. The pulses, which are felt on the wrist when diagnosing an imbalance, are Yang or husband on the left wrist, and Yin or wife on the right. Because the male is dominant, the pulse on the left wrist must be stronger, and the acupuncturist must be careful not to upset this balance.

3. The Noon-Midnight Law. Certain organs are best treated at certain times of the day. The day is divided thus:

Midnight – 2 a.m.	Gall Bladder.
2 a.m. – 4 a.m.	Liver.
4 a.m. – 6 a.m.	Lungs.
6 a.m. – 8 a.m.	Large Intestine.
8 a.m. – 10 a.m.	Stomach.
10 a.m. – 12 noon.	Spleen.

Noon – 2 p.m.	Heart.
2 p.m. – 4 p.m.	Small Intestine.
4 p.m. – 6 p.m.	Bladder.
6 p.m. – 8 p.m.	Kidneys.
8 p.m. – 10 p.m.	Circulation or Sex.
10 p.m. – midnight	Triple Warmer.

Stimulation of an organ on this chart will also stimulate the organ in the time division twelve hours later. So stimulation of the Gall Bladder meridian would also stimulate the Heart meridian. It will be clear from the chart at what times of the day the various meridians are best stimulated, and hence a patient's treatment will be governed by the time of his consultation, and appointments organised according to the best time to treat him.

It is interesting to compare this with the findings of western researchers recorded in "The Body Clock Diet" by Ronald Gatty (Gollancz 1980). This book uses the rhythms of the body mainly as an aid to diet, of course, but it does look at the cycles, which are not only daily, but weekly and monthly. We all know, to give a simple example, that there are times when we are accident prone.

4. The Law of the Five Elements. We have already looked briefly at the interaction of one meridian on another, paralleling the interaction of the elements in nature. This last of the four laws sets out this interaction as follows:

Water creates wood but destroys fire.
Wood creates fire but destroys earth.
Fire creates earth but destroys metal.
Earth creates metal but destroys water.
Metal creates water but destroys wood.

This, translated into the interactions of the corresponding meridians, becomes:

Kidney meridian increases liver meridian but
    decreases heart.
Liver meridian increases heart but decreases
    spleen.
Heart meridian increases spleen but decreases lung.

Spleen meridian increases lung but decreases
kidney.
Lung meridian increases kidney but decreases liver.

To stimulate either Yin or Yang in a meridian, the acupuncturist inserts his needle rapidly and withdraws it slowly, massaging the spot afterwards. To calm Yin or Yang, he does the same thing, but does not massage the spot afterwards. The only difference between treating Yin and Yang in this respect is that for Yin he uses cold needles and for Yang he uses hot ones. Twisting the needle clockwise when it is inserted will stimulate Yang, and twisting it anti-clockwise will stimulate Yin. The time the needle must be left in is determined by feeling the patient's pulse, and this brings us to a very important part of the acupuncturist's technique.

Diagnosis is always made or confirmed by taking the pulse. An irregular pulse indicates that something is wrong; once the needles have regularised it, they can be withdrawn, because balance has been restored. Western doctors say that there is only one pulse, and that it is only of limited help in diagnosis. Often, the regular taking of it will be left to a junior nurse in hospital, and the doctor will simply note if it is high or low in rate. The acupuncturist, on the other hand, claims to feel twelve separate pulses, and from these, that he can detect exactly what is wrong. Other symptoms of the patient may be misleading, but the pulses are never wrong.

The acupuncturist will therefore spend anything from ten minutes to a couple of hours taking his patient's pulse. He places the tips of his first three fingers on the radial artery at about the same place that the Western doctor or nurse does, but with each finger he is feeling a different pulse. The section nearest the patient's wrist is known as the "inch"; the next section is the "bar"; the section furthest from the hand is called the "cubit". The patient is always asked to sit quietly or even to lie down for about ten minutes before the pulse is taken, and the acupuncturist will in this time take his own pulse, so that he can consider the effect of this on his diagnosis.

If the patient is a man, the acupuncturist will take his left wrist first; if a woman, her right wrist. At first, he feels the pulses lightly, and this, he claims, reveals the three superficial pulses in each wrist. On the right wrist, these superficial pulses give a guide to the large intestine (by the inch), the stomach (by the bar), and the Triple Warmer (by the cubit). On the left wrist, these superficial pulses give a guide to the small intestine (by the inch), the gall bladder (by the bar), and the bladder (by the cubit).

Having taken these superficial pulses in each wrist, the acupuncturist will now press a little harder on the wrist, and claims he will then be able to feel deeper pulses. On the right wrist, these deeper pulses give indications to the lungs (by the inch), the spleen (by the bar), and the circulation-sex meridian (by the cubit). On the left wrist, the deeper indications are the heart (by the inch), the liver (by the bar), and the kidneys (by the cubit). Not only is the acupuncturist able to feel and to distinguish these twelve pulses, three deep and three superficial on each wrist, he also claims to be able to sense twenty-seven different qualities in each of them. Each quality is a guide to a specific illness.

Added to all this, he must consider that the pulses will naturally be stronger in Summer than in Spring, and that they will wane in the Autumn, and be deep in the Winter. If the pulses are too hard, too much Ch'i is present in one organ or another, and he must use his needles to restore the balance of Yin and Yang.

By this method of pulse diagnosis, Chinese masters claim to be able to detect illness before any other symptoms are visible, and even to predict future illnesses a year or two hence. Some also believe they can foretell the sex of an unborn child. In ancient times, Chinese doctors were forbidden to look on the form of a woman, and pulse diagnosis plus questioning was the only way they could find out what was wrong with her. Over the centuries, it has developed into a highly skilled art.

In people whose pulses are very weak, such as the chronically sick or very young children, the acupuncturist will have to base his diagnosis on three other methods: inspecting the patient, hearing, and smelling. He will be trained to observe subtle changes in a patient's skin which can betoken illness; the eyes will indicate liver complaints or disorders of the spleen or lungs; the tongue will reveal kidney ailments. Changes in a patient's voice, rasping breath, and different body odours also give tell-tale signs to the expert who can read them.

Having decided where to use his needles, the acupuncturist must decide which needle. He has nine different ones. The chisel needle has an end like an arrow head and is used for treating skin complaints; the needle with the rounded end is used to massage muscles; the spoon needle is used when the pulses are strong; the lance needle is rarely used; the stiletto needle which is shaped like a curved sword is used only in chronic cases; the round sharp needle relieves pain and paralytic conditions; the long soft hair needle, which is often plunged in to its full length, relieves numbness and pain; the seven inch needle relieves deep pain; and the fire needle is used in cases of poisoning and swelling.

In the early days, these needles were made of silver or gold or sometimes of copper or brass. Even earlier ones made of flint have been found. Today, however, needles are invariably made of stainless steel. Often only one treatment with them is required, since according to the philosophy of the art, all that is needed for recovery is to restore the balance of Yin and Yang, and thus bring the patient back into harmony with the Universe.

Perhaps the application of acupuncture that is best known in the West is its use as an anaesthetic. When President Nixon of the United States made his visit to China, this use of acupuncture attracted considerable publicity in the United States and in Britain. By inserting a needle at the correct point and twirling it, all sensation of pain could apparently be removed, and patients would lie awake and even talk to their surgeons during quite severe operations. Sometimes the twirling by hand was replaced by passing a small electric current through the needle. Sheets would be pulled up to prevent the patient seeing what was being done to him, of course, since even in the most hardy, this could produce shock. But patients have still been quite happy under this anaesthesia, and the after-effect of the drugs normally given is completely lacking. Healing is said to be quicker on this account. Amongst other operations that have been carried out in this way are removal of appendix, heart and lung surgery. Any one of these would result in unbearable pain, if the needle technique did not work. Even dentists use this technique in China. One needle inserted between the thumb and the first finger enables teeth to be extracted with no other anaesthetic.

One other technique that acupuncturists use is moxa-bustion. This is the burning of a small pile of moxa, which is the leaf of the Chinese wormwood tree, either on the skin, or on a little attachment on the head of a needle. If on the skin, it is done after the needle is withdrawn; if on the needle, it results in a hot needle. This technique cannot be used on all acupuncture points, indeed it is dangerous on some of them, so its use is restricted to comparatively few treatments.

Of recent years, acupuncture has spread to Europe and to the Soviet Union, and a great deal of public interest has been aroused. Remarkable cures have been claimed for the treatment. In 1966, at the Peking Hospital, 151 patients paralysed from the waist down were treated; three years after, 124 of them could walk unaided. Another success has been claimed with deaf children. The treatment in this case required the repeated insertion of the needles just behind the ears. Polio, epileptic seizures, and depression have all been successfully treated with acupuncture. The main areas where it cannot be used are accidents and surgical emergencies and those diseases which are transmitted by bacteria. Some of the latter were unknown in China until Western traders went there, and this fact probably delayed research into the possible measures that could be taken against them.

Acupressure is the technique of putting pressure on the acupuncture spots with the fingers instead of inserting needles. It is often used on sensitive patients, and on those who fear the needles, though it should be said that the needles do not hurt, and the patient will feel them far less than a hypodermic injection; indeed, if he shuts his eyes, he may not feel them at all.

Acu*pressure* is often used by patients for self-treatment, when they have learnt the techniques. It will relieve pain, help in the case of insomnia, and aid dieting, to give three simple examples. You can experiment on yourself without danger, and find what kind of pressure relieves what kind of pain. As one example, to press hard on the fleshy part between thumb and forefinger will relieve toothache. This is the very point at which the dentist would insert a needle if he were doing an extraction without anaesthetic. Pressure at the same point will also relieve constipation, period pains, and headache. There is a point on the inside of the lip which will reduce appetite. There are points on the forehead, wrist and the inside of the leg for insomnia. I have seen nose bleeding stopped by pressure on the hand. There are books on the subject for those who wish to use these simple therapies on themselves, or acupuncturists can show their patients what to do.

The first question most people will ask about acupuncture is, can it help me? In the case of migraine, headaches, allergies, rheumatism, arthritis, depression, or in childbirth, the answer is almost certainly, Yes. In 1979, the World Health Organisation listed the diseases that responded best to acupuncture treatment. As well as the above, they included sinusitis, the common cold, tonsilitis, bronchitis, asthma, eye disorders, toothache, gastritis, colitis, duodenal ulcers, constipation, diarrhoea, and Menière's disease.

Any reputable acupuncturist will tell you frankly whether he can help you or not. He will not use his needles unless he thinks they are going to do some good. He has his reputation to consider.

The next question people ask is, does it hurt?, and particularly in a book on Healing without Harm, this is a relevant consideration. The simple answer is, No. Some patients report a slight burning sensation, some a rush of energy. To reassure the sensitive, the practitioner will often demonstrate by sticking a needle into his own body first, but if you are still nervous you could ask for acupressure instead. The only drawback is that the treatment being milder the effect is likely to be less effective than the needles.

After treatment, some patients feel tired and need to rest; others, on the contrary feel more alert. Reactions differ. One treatment may be all that is needed for some conditions; some will require more; still others will be helped by regular treatment over a period of time, so that not only are the patient's energies restored to harmony, but they are maintained in that state. This can be a form of preventive medicine.

The final question is, where do I go for treatment?

In Britain, you can obtain registers of qualified acupuncturists for a small fee from one of the colleges that train them. See the Appendix page 148 for their addresses.

Some acupuncturists have no other medical qualification, but this does not mean that they are necessarily less skilled. Some who are medically qualified may have taken only a short course in acupuncture abroad. Of course, there are charlatans with no qualifications at all. It is worth trying to find out where the person you consult was trained, and being wary of those who are reluctant to say.

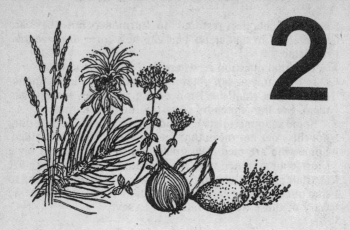

2

AROMA THERAPY

Aroma therapy uses aromatic essences from plants to treat diseases and as a preventive measure against disease. It is by no means a modern concept; the Egyptians used myrrh and cinnamon to embalm the dead as long ago as 4500 B.C.; the Good Samaritan in the Bible treated the man who fell among thieves with oil and wine; the Greeks knew the value of the onion plant; aromatic herbs were used in fighting the 14th century Plague known as The Black Death.

In the First World War, dozens of doctors were re-discovering the value of essences in helping wounds to heal, and in the 1930's, Dr. René Maurice Gattefossé, a Frenchman, published a comprehensive book on aroma therapy. Still more recently, another Frenchman, Jean Valnet, has contributed to the growing acceptance of the treatment. With more and more people turning away from the use of drugs today, aroma therapy is becoming more popular.

One drawback to the use of conventional synthetic drugs,

which is often overlooked both by patients and by the doctors who prescribe them, is the fact that the body comes to tolerate them. And they are then no longer as effective. The traditional remedy for this is to prescribe larger doses or new drugs, but it becomes a vicious circle. As we have mentioned earlier in this book, drugs can set up allergies, or have side-effects which are at the least unpleasant and at the worst dangerous and maiming. None of these dangers exists with aroma therapy, though of course dosage is important, and even with plant remedies an overdose can be harmful.

The essences used in aroma therapy are usually obtained from the plants by distillation, and they are generally prescribed in the form of drops or capsules by a doctor who uses aroma therapy as part of his treatment. The oils are also used by modern aromatherapists to massage the body either in a particular area or by a general method known as "the lymphatic drainage massage technique" at which we shall look later on. Simply using some of the plants, such as garlic, thyme, sage and cloves, in the kitchen as seasoning has a beneficial effect, and the essences can be added to baths, made up into liniments or infusions or soups, or used for fumigation. Sometimes, too, the patient will sprinkle a few drops into a bowl of boiling water, and inhale the aroma. The best inhalations for head cold are six drops of eucalyptus to two drops of peppermint and two drops of basil. For influenza, seven drops of eucalyptus, three of camphor and two of black pepper. For bronchitis, four drops of eucalyptus, four of bergamot and four of sandalwood. All these usages form part of aroma therapy.

Because very little of an essence is obtained by distillation from a plant, the process is laborious and the cost of the essences is high, but against this can be set the fact that very small doses are needed to get results. In this, aroma-therapists would agree with homoeopaths that often the smaller the dose the greater the effect, though, of course, aromatherapists do not use the minute traces that homoeo-opaths do.

Some plants will yield their essences by other methods, such as pressing or tapping, heating, or the use of solvents. Obviously it is in their pure form that the essences are most effective, and plants from certain localities are better than the same plants from other areas. Some of the oils marketed commercially may be adulterated, and patients who are treating themselves should consider this possibility, and purchase with care.

Aromatic essences have an antiseptic use. In sprays they are more potent than synthetic preparations when used against germs in the air. Lemon, thyme, orange, bergamot, juniper, clove, peppermint, rosemary, sandalwood and eucalyptus are all used for this purpose. It is claimed that cloves will kill the tuberculosis bacillus in the air and lemon will destroy typhus bacillus, pneumococcus and meningococcus.

The essences can be used in solutions to treat wounds and have a rapid healing effect that compares favourably with synthetic drugs because they are harmless to tissue. Chemical antiseptics can be as harmful to the cells of the body with which they come into contact as to the microbes they are battling with.

It has been found that if aromatic essences are used in baths, the body will absorb them through the pores as well as by breathing in the vapours, so that benefit is derived in both these ways as well as by the local action on the skin itself. Essences absorbed in this way go right into the internal organs.

As examples of the use of aroma therapy, we find that influenza responds to treatment by cinnamon, pine needles, thyme, and lemon; gangrenous wounds frequently respond to lavender; scabies to lavender, lemon, rosemary, orange-flower, mustard, and thyme; insect pests can be repelled or their bites soothed by lavender, geranium and origanum. In this latter case, rubbing the bitten area with the flowers of lavender, the leaves of sage, or a cut leek or onion will cause the pain to disappear and the inflammation to subside. It is thought that broom neutralises adder venom, since sheep which feed on broom are resistant to their bites. Rheumatism can be helped by compresses of garlic, onion, thyme, or sage. Even to eat a clove of garlic a day will help rheumatic patients.

Taken internally, essences are even more powerful than

when used externally. The use of essential oils in the treatment of tuberculosis lowers temperature, reduces coughing, and leads to increased weight and strength. Tarragon oil can be taken to stop hiccoughs. There is some controversy, however, as to whether the oils should be taken internally. Some practitioners feel that they are too strong and that the mucous membrane of the digestive tract is particularly sensitive to them. Certainly their internal use does not combine with some other forms of medication and their use in this way should only be on the advice of a doctor. Essences which have a stimulating effect are: pine needles, geranium, basil, sage, aniseed, mint, onion, garlic and lemon. Essences which have a sedative effect are: nutmeg, lavender, and bergamot.

The technique of lymphatic drainage massage referred to earlier uses oils to penetrate the skin and hence the whole body system. The therapist starts massaging the patient's legs and his back to push all the accumulated toxins in his body up the lymphatic system. He then goes on to massage the head, face, chest and arms, with the result that all the poisons end up in the area of the groin, where they will be naturally evacuated. Ideally this form of massage should be done once a week by a trained therapist, and the patient will feel renewed and refreshed.

Patients can undertake general massage of their own bodies of course, and for this purpose the following mixtures of oil should be used: for muscles and general aches, ten drops of juniper and five of rosemary in a vegetable oil solution; for rheumatism, seven drops of eucalyptus, seven of camphor and seven of rosemary, in a vegetable oil solution; for relaxation, ten drops of geranium, seven of lavender and four of marjoram, again in a vegetable oil solution.

Many of the remedies used in aroma therapy have been known in folklore for generations. The herbs used in the preparation of food in tropical countries such as the curry powders have their uses in destroying any germs in the food. Onion has always been used in folk medicine as a cure for colds. Hot onion broth is a well-known country remedy, which today is sometimes being recommended for prostate conditions. Ginseng is just now becoming popular in the West as a tonic and a reported aphrodisiac. Burns were regularly treated by country folk with a mixture of herb essences used as a poultice. I can recall a chopped-up raw potato being used with good effect in my own case. The time taken for the skin to heal with any of these treatments is lessened. Herb pillows are another example of aroma therapy. They are a favourite way of inducing restful sleep, and if a few drops of cypress are sprinkled on an ordinary pillow spasmodic coughing can be controlled. Sanatoria for chest complaints are usually located in the country and often amid pine-covered hills, as the aroma is believed to be beneficial.

Aroma therapy does not claim to be able to cure every ill. In fact it is a treatment usually used in conjunction with other medical treatments. It is, however, holistic in approach, and the aromatherapist will, before he begins treatment, take time to find out all about the patient. He will want to delve into past medical history, hereditary ailments, the kind of food the patient eats, the amount of exercise he takes, weight, any other medicines he is taking, his work including any stresses he encounters in that work, family life, hobbies, indeed beliefs. From all this information the therapist can build up a complete picture of the patient in his environment, and this will enable him to prescribe the essences and treatments needed to help the condition which the patient is currently complaining of.

The therapist will have the wider aim of improving the patient's overall health, however. As well as baths or massage or doses of suitable oils, diet changes and exercise may be prescribed. All these will help the patient to fight off his present disease but they will also make him less vulnerable in the future.

France is much more advanced than Britain in the practice of aroma therapy. Belgium and Russia are developing the practice, and the United States is beginning to show interest. Usually therapists have normal medical training and then take a post-graduate course in aroma therapy. Such courses are available for doctors in Britain at The College of Natural Therapies (for the address see the Appendix page 148). The college also runs courses for those who are not medically qualified. These students take a diploma, and will normally carry out massage, prescribe baths and diet. Qualified doctors will make a normal diagnosis and may treat by conventional methods or by aroma therapy or by a combination of both.

When should you consult an aromatherapist? As has already been indicated, nearly every condition except those requiring urgent surgery can be helped, and even in surgical cases, the wounds can be helped to heal more quickly if aroma therapy is used. Cancer is said sometimes to respond though not by any means in all cases. The oils have antiseptic qualities, and in all cases they will combat infection. They act as diuretics; they help rheumatism, they are effective with circulatory troubles, and they help the nervous system. We all know from experience that a pleasant fragrance is refreshing in the case of anxiety or depression. It makes us feel better, and that is a first step towards being better.

There is no condition that is without a herbal remedy. To list only a few will encourage those who are interested to enquire further. Pain responds to aniseed, camomile, and clove. Cancer can sometimes be helped by clove, cypress, garlic, onion, and sage. Diabetes by eucalyptus, geranium, juniper and onion. Gallstones by lemon, onion and pine. Infections by camphor, clove, eucalyptus, and garlic. Influenza by eucalyptus, garlic, lemon, peppermint and thyme. Malaria by eucalyptus and lemon. Obesity by lemon and onion. Arthritis by onion, pine and sage. Stones in the urine by fennel, garlic, geranium, hyssop and lemon. Healing of wounds by clove, eucalyptus, garlic, geranium, hyssop, sage, lemon and thyme. Prostate troubles by onion, thuja and thyme. Nerves by basil, cypress, lavender, marjoram, and rosemary. The circulation by carraway, cinnamon, garlic and nutmeg. The digestive organs by aniseed, carraway, cinnamon, fennel, garlic, and onion. The pancreas by lemon. Respiratory disorders by aniseed, cinnamon, and garlic.

No-one should treat themselves from the above list however. There are many other remedies, and a trained therapist or a doctor specialising in aroma therapy should be consulted. He will prescribe the exact remedy for your condition, possibly in conjunction with some other medication. For example, a diabetic cannot simply give up insulin and resort to aroma therapy. All that he can hope is that properly prescribed doses of aroma therapy will reduce the dosage of insulin he needs over a period of time, and of course the process must be medically monitored.

The only self-help anyone should contemplate in this field of healing is dietary improvement, regular exercise, experimenting with oils in the normal baths, and occasionally special baths, such as salt baths for cleansing. A good soak for ten minutes or so will do much to ease away your aches and pains.

The main dietary changes that should be considered are: replacing tea and coffee with herbal teas; replacing full cream milk with skim milk or fruit juice; eating as many salads as possible; using organically grown vegetables; choosing fish rather than meat as the main protein source.

Relaxation should be practised of course. Stress and tension work against improvement in health, and this is where relaxing baths come into their own.

If you wish to consult an aromatherapist, you can get a list from the various associations mentioned in the Appendix page 148. Practitioners' announcements appear regularly in the magazine "Here's Health", though you should note that medically qualified therapists do not advertise. There are several clinics in London, and one in Ashtead, Surrey (The Vera Schonberg Health and Beauty Clinic).

Treatment at a clinic tends to be expensive, however, and if all you want is to try a few drops of oil in your bath, you can buy the oils from the suppliers mentioned in the Appendix page 149.

You can either put combinations straight into your bath, or you can prepare combinations to keep by you, to use for the different purposes. If you are mixing straight into the bath, try:

Two drops of basil, four of geranium and two of hyssop for
    nervous exhaustion;
Two drops of camomile, five of lavender and two of orange
    blossom for a sedative;

Two drops of fennel, two of rosemary and four of juniper for a hangover;

Five drops of rosemary, five of juniper and five of peppermint to give you energy in the morning.

If you want to prepare mixtures to keep by you, make the following mixtures, and when you need them use from two to eight drops in a bath filled with warm water:

Lavender (5 drops), cypress (5 drops), marjoram (4 drops), camomile (2 drops), orange blossom (2 drops) and rose (2 drops) will provide a relaxing mix;

Rosemary (5 drops), juniper (5 drops), hyssop (3 drops), peppermint (3 drops), and basil (3 drops) will stimulate you.

Lavender (5 drops), juniper (5 drops), cypress (5 drops), geranium (4 drops), lemon (4 drops) peppermint (4 drops) and bergamot (3 drops) will refresh you;

And, for a sensual bath, try sandalwood (8 drops), ylang-ylang (3 drops), orange blossom (2 drops) and jasmine (2 drops).

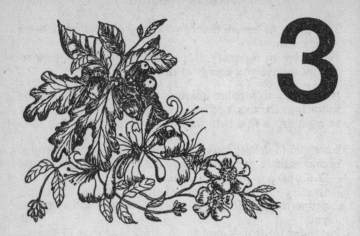

3

BACH FLOWER REMEDIES

The system of treatment by the Bach Flower Remedies was discovered by Dr. Edward Bach, a famous physician who practised in Harley Street for over twenty years. He was greatly impressed with the work of Hahnemann in homoeopathy, and discovered the healing power of flowers. In 1930, he gave up his practice to devote all his time to finding the remedies that were most effective and to perfecting the method of using them. Originally, there were twelve remedies, listed in his book "The Twelve Healers". Living in the country and walking the fields, he gradually discovered others by experiment and by the sensitivity he developed to the effects and the moods of people. Eventually, he added another twenty-six remedies to the original ones making thirty-eight in all.

The basis of Dr. Bach's system was his belief that illness is the result of a conflict between the soul of man and the mind. Because it had this spiritual base, illness could never be cured by purely materialistic means. To take a simple example, we all know that worry or fear will lower our vitality and impede our recovery, and conversely that if we get rid of the worry or fear, our body will be in a better position to heal itself or to resist any infection to which we may be exposed.

This is the idea behind all Dr. Bach's treatments. The remedies are prescribed not for a particular complaint, but according to the personality or moods of the patient. Dr. Bach said: "They cure, not by attacking the disease, but by flooding our. bodies with the beautiful vibrations of our Higher Nature, in the presence of which disease melts away as snow in the sunshine."

The thirty-eight remedies can be used in conjunction with other methods of treatment, though naturopathic doctors or homoeopaths are more likely to be sympathetic to their use than orthodox medical practitioners who would view them rather as they view homoeopathy. They can also be used for self-treatment by those who have the objectivity to observe their own personality traits. Those for whom such objectivity is difficult would be better advised to consult a healer skilled in the Bach method.

There is no mystery about the preparation of the remedies. If you have the time and the skill to recognise the flowers needed, you can prepare the basic stock. Gather the flowers when they are in full bloom. Fill a shallow dish with one pint of the purest water available, spring or well water being preferred to tap water; rain water can be used, but not distilled water. Float the blooms on the water so that they cover the entire surface, and leave in bright sunlight for three to four hours or until the flowers start to fade. Pour the liquid into bottles with equal parts of brandy. This makes your basic stock, as it is called. Dilute this by using five drops of the liquid with one fluid ounce of water. Bottle this and seal it, and you have the remedy you are going to use.

With flowers and twigs that bloom very early in the year, before the sun reaches its full intensity, you can prepare the remedies by boiling the flowers gently for half an hour, then filtering off the liquid and mixing it with the appropriate measure of brandy.

If you do not wish to prepare your own remedies or distrust your ability, you can buy them from some chemists or direct from The Dr. Edward Bach Centre (see the Appendix page 149 for the address). This was Dr. Bach's home and the flowers used in the preparation there are growing in the same areas that he found the original ones. You can buy the remedies singly or as a complete set of thirty-eight. You can also buy them made up into a grease-less ointment with a homoeopathic base, and the centre has a variety of excellent and inexpensive books on the subject, which will give you far more detailed information than is possible in a chapter of this kind. Treatment is also available at the centre.

The remedies are usually taken by mouth, but they can be used as a lotion or compress or hot fomentation, or they can be added to a bath. The normal dose is five drops in a tablespoonful of water, two or three times a day, but you can take them oftener if you need. They are quite harmless and there is no fear of over-dosing.

If you seek treatment from a practitioner, he will encourage you to talk about yourself and your problems, because he is not basically concerned with the physical condition that drives you to seek his help but with what kind of person you are and with your emotional state. You should talk quite freely with him, because he is not there to judge or condemn you, but to help you. He will learn a lot about you from your behaviour and your appearance and even from the tone of your voice, because often these things are more revealing than what you say. He will help you to face your inner feelings, things you would not normally admit to yourself or reveal to others, because facing up to these truths is a big step towards a cure.

If you decide after reading the books on the subject that you feel you can prescribe for yourself, you must have this same honesty in facing your feelings. Consider how you behave when you are very tired, or in a serious emergency, if you have to make an important decision, or if the weather is gloomy. Are you easily irritated by other people? Are you depressed about life, seeing no hope? Do you harbour feelings of hatred, envy or jealousy? Do you suffer from guilt? Do you find it difficult to make decisions? Do you look back with longing to a happy past, or with anger to an unhappy past? Do you have fears, and if so, are they fears of something in particular or of some vague nameless disaster or horror? Are you serene in an emergency or do you get flustered? Do you have problems in your work or in your home? Answer these questions honestly, and try to confirm your answers by consulting someone you trust and who knows you well enough to speak frankly with you. When you have the answers, you will have no difficulty in seeing which remedy meets your condition, and as you start to treat yourself for the kind of person you are, so any illness you have will begin to show an improvement.

Children and even babies can be treated by the Bach remedies. You have only to observe them. Indeed it is often easier to prescribe for a child or a baby than for an adult, because they have not learnt to hide their emotions. Babies will be fretful or contented; distressed by the absence of those they love; screaming for attention or unduly placid; easily frightened or indifferent; too active or needing too much sleep. Discover the type of child or baby you are dealing with rather than concentrate on particular physical symptoms, though of course consult a doctor if these give cause for alarm.

Animals and plants also benefit from the Bach remedies. Each animal is an individual. Your dog or your cat has a personality of its own of which you may already be aware. They may be frightened, angry, impatient, or dreamy. It is only recently that feelings have been ascribed to plants with any scientific foundation. They can however show susceptibility to love or anger. They can suffer from shock, as when they are transplanted or pruned. To treat animals, put the dose in their food, or rub it around their lips so that they will lick it off. For plants, put two drops of each remedy you are giving in a bottle, then use one teaspoonful of the mixture to one gallon of water, and make a spray to go round the base of the plant.

More than one remedy can be taken at once, and they can be varied according to progress. The usual practice is to decide on the basic type of the patient, and to include this remedy in all the doses, and then to add extra remedies for any temporary condition. For example, you will easily diagnose a self-centred possessive type of patient as being a "chicory" type. Then, if he had changing moods or difficulty in making decisions, you would add scleranthus. If he was in despair, feeling that the remedy was not doing any good, you would add gentian. Later, the despondency might give way to confidence and hope, and the gentian could be omitted.

The thirty-eight remedies, and the types of people they may help are as follows:

1. Agrimony (*Agrimonia eupatoria*)

Agrimony is for the type who suffer worries that may amount to mental torture, but which they hide from other people, so that they may appear quite care-free on the surface. They will make light of any illness in conversation; they will seek companionship as an escape from their worries. They may suffer insomnia but they will not talk about it. In severe cases they may resort to drink or drugs to calm their anxieties.

2. Aspen (*Populus tremula*)

Aspen is for the type who suffers from vague fears. Because the fear is vague and cannot be given a name, this type of person will usually try to hide their fear from others and to battle with it alone. If it were something specific like a visit to the doctor or the dentist, they might cope with it better, or at least share it, but usually it comes from sources such as a bad dream that they cannot quite remember on waking, or sometimes from thoughts of death or religion.

3. Beech (*Fagus sylvatica*)

Beech is for the intolerant person, who does not even try to understand other people or to make allowances for their shortcomings. Such people are very critical and see only the faults in other people. Often quite trivial mannerisms or gestures will annoy out of all proportion to their significance, and this intolerance makes beech people very lonely and isolated individuals.

4. Centaury (*Centaurium umbellatum*)

Centaury is for the type who is weak-willed. Centaury types are quiet timid people who are easily influenced by others. They are willing to be used by other people, and often become "doormats" for more dominant personalities, ill-used and over-worked, because they do not have the strength of will to stand up for themselves. Often they are mentally very alert and active, but this will not show. They appear pale and languid, because of the drain on them arising from the way they are put upon.

5. Cerato (*Ceratostigma millmottiana*)

Cerato is for people who doubt their own ability and get led by others against their better judgment, even though they themselves are wise intuitive people with very definite opinions of their own. Because of their distrust of their own judgment, they tend to seek advice of all and sundry when a decision has to be made, and often they will follow this advice when their own better judgment would tell them otherwise. Normally they will be very talkative people, and they often get led astray into foolish behaviour.

6. Cherry Plum (*Prunus cerasifera*)

Cherry plum is for the type who get driven into such a state of desperation that they fear they will lose control of their mind and do some dreadful thing. They are afraid they will be driven to doing physical injury to someone who irritates them, or that they will go mad and run beserk. Often they are on the verge of a nervous breakdown. They may even contemplate suicide.

7. Chestnut Bud (*Aesculus hippocastanum*)

Chestnut bud is for the type who makes the same mistake over and over again, failing to learn by experience. Their errors may be due to hurry, indifference, inattention or lack of observation, but because they are always trying to forget the past, they do not have this reservoir of experience to guide them in the future.

8. Chicory (*Cichorium intybus*)

Chicory is for the self-centred possessive type. They are full of self-love and self-pity. They tend to nag and to control the lives of others, even of those for whom they care. If they cannot get their own way, they fret, and make martyrs of themselves in their own eyes. A typical reaction is to simulate illness in order to keep relatives subservient to them and to get attention.

9. Clematis (*Clematis vitalba*)

Clematis is for the dreamy absent-minded type who may appear indifferent to what is going on. They live in their thoughts, and withdraw into the private world of their dreams in order to escape from the unpleasant realities of life. They have poor memories because their thoughts are far away and they do not concentrate on what is going on. Sometimes they will fail to recognise people they know in the street. When ill, they will often make no real effort to get well. They sometimes become willing partners to a suicide pact, because they would rather die with a loved one than survive alone.

10. Crab Apple (*Malus sylvestris*)

Crab apple is for the type who feel they need cleansing. They may be over-sensitive to the point of disgust with themselves over some trivial blemish such as a wart or a rash. It may be some quality of their behaviour which disgusts them. They concentrate on these trivial matters to the exclusion of more important things, and will frequently suffer from despondency that may deepen into despair.

11. Elm (*Ulmus procera*)

Elm is for the type who are very capable, who know their own capabilities, but who at times become exhausted by their striving for perfection, and who in such times will feel inadequate and wonder how they are going to carry on. They quite often hold positions of importance in the community. Their exhaustion leads to despondency, but it is always a temporary condition because they have an inner conviction that the work they have chosen to do in life is their vocation, and they believe in their hearts that they will be given the strength to see it through.

12. Gentian (*Gentiana amarella*),

Gentian is for the type who suffers from deep depression leading to melancholia. They are people who are easily discouraged by set-backs, even though there are specific and known causes for these set-backs. They find it hard to be happy even when things are going well, and are pessimistic. They do not understand that often it is their own attitude that leads to things going wrong, and that certainly makes everything seem so much worse when they do go wrong.

13. Gorse (*Ulex europaeus*)

Gorse is for the type of person who has lost heart and knows the despair that utter hopelessness brings. Perhaps they suffer from an illness for which they have tried many remedies, none of which has worked, and now they are resigned to suffering for the rest of their lives. Perhaps it is not a physical illness but a condition of life that they cannot find a remedy for. Sometimes they become convinced that hereditary factors are responsible.

14. Heather (*Calluna vulgaris*)

Heather is for the self-centred types who, unlike the chicory types, are not also full of self-pity. They are however full of the problems, the ailments, and all the trivial things of their own lives, to the exclusion of all else. They dislike being alone because they want an audience for their woes. They always want to be the centre of interest in a conversation, and are poor listeners, since they have little interest in other people.

15. Holly (*Ilex aquifolium*)

Holly is for the type who is filled with hatred, envy, jealousy or suspicion. Dr. Bach saw this as a root cause of evil, since these feelings are the opposite of the love that should unite man to his fellows and to God. Hatred breeds insecurity, aggressiveness and anger. These are all negative qualities and hurt the person who suffers them even more than the person against whom they are directed. Dr. Bach said that holly was the most important of the remedies because it "protects us from all that is not Universal Love".

16. Honeysuckle (*Lonicera caprifolium*)

Honeysuckle is for the type who dwells in the past. It is for those who hark back to their happy memories of childhood. It is for those who are homesick. It is equally for those whose memories are unhappy, such as a soldier with terrible war experiences behind him. In all such cases, the reversion to the past leads to a lack of interest in the present, and to a slowing down of life's processes.

17. Hornbeam (*Carpinus betulus*)

Hornbeam is for the type who suffers from continual tiredness. Often it is a mental state rather than physical exhaustion. They feel that they do not have the strength to go on, but that they would have if they could overcome this feeling. When convalescent after an illness, they will wonder if they will ever regain their strength even though doctors can assure them they are on the mend. Even in health they feel tired. Getting up in the morning will always be a burden.

18. Impatiens (*Impatiens glandulifera*)

Impatiens is for the type who is very active, nervous and impatient. They make instant decisions themselves and are very good and efficient at whatever they do, but they easily become irritated with those who are slower. They are quick to become angry, though their anger subsides just as quickly. Because of their irritability and because they eat too quickly, they are prone to digestive complaints.

19. Larch (*Larix decidua*)

Larch is for the type of person who lacks confidence in himself. They are normally people who are quite capable and indeed who are often superior in ability to their fellows, but because they have no faith in their ability, they anticipate failure and often are led into despair. They are never envious of another's success, nor are they frightened people; it is just that they will seldom attempt anything because they feel sure they will fail.

20. Mimulus (*Mimulus guttatus*)

Mimulus is for the person who is afraid but who knows what he is afraid of, unlike the aspen type whose fears have no name. Mimulus types may fear pain or death. They may fear something like speaking in public. Stage fright will then cause them to blush and stammer. They are always shy and retiring people, but they are a type who can be especially helped by the flower remedies, because mimulus can cure them once and for all.

21. Mustard (*Sinapis arvenis*)

Mustard is for the person on whom black depression or gloom will settle for no apparent reason. The depression will shut out all his joy in living and turn his thoughts in on himself, so that he is not normal. This condition may last a day or so, and usually lifts of its own accord, but the cause of the bout of melancholia is never known. Mustard will help.

22. Oak (*Quercus robur*)

Oak is for the type whose despondency is of a different

kind. It is for people who struggle on in the face of adversity never giving up hope. Physically oak types are strong. They are patient and full of common sense, but sometimes despair can become too much for them, and they will crack up and suffer a nervous breakdown.

23. Olive (*Olea europaea*)

Olive is for those whose strength has been sapped by long suffering under either illness or adversity. Physically and mentally they have reached a state of complete exhaustion. Olive is helpful in convalescence or in the case of those people who lead such full lives they have no time for rest or recreation.

24. Pine (*Pinus sylvestris*)

Pine is for those who suffer from feelings of guilt leading to self-reproach. They are over-conscientious. They set themselves very high standards and are in despair when they fail to live up to them. They never blame others when things go wrong, but always themselves. They develop guilt complexes about such things as living in comfort when so many in the world are without necessities.

25. Red Chestnut (*Aesculus carnea*)

Red chestnut is for the type who is fearful for others. Their fears become a perpetual anxiety. If their loved ones are late home in the evening, or if they do not hear from them immediately they have arrived after a journey, they will fear the worst. If someone near to them has a minor ailment they will fear that it could become a major illness. These fears do not of course help the person about whom they are worrying; indeed their fears may be transferred to the object of their anxiety.

26. Rock Rose (*Helianthemum chamaecistus*)

Rock rose is for those who suffer terror or panic. They may be victims of an accident; they may simply have witnessed an accident. Even nightmares may produce the kind of terror they feel. It is interesting to note that terror in people around may produce terror in this type of person, even though he did not originally feel it himself, and thus the kind of anxiety of the red chestnut type does nothing to help the rock rose type.

27. Rock Water

Rock water is not a flower; it is simply pure water from the rocks. It is for those who are as hard as a rock, and the theory is that as water will wear away a rock, so the remedy will wear away the sufferer's insensibility and inflexible nature. The type of person who may benefit are those who hold strong views on religion or politics amounting perhaps to bigotry, though they do not usually try to force their views on others. They simply set themselves high ideals which they force themselves to live up to, often becoming martyrs in the attempt. They are like the old hermits who would "mortify the flesh" for spiritual ends.

28. Scleranthus (*Scleranthus annuus*)

Scleranthus is for the type of person who cannot make up his mind. Such people hesitate and dither; they jump from one thing to another; they suffer extremes of joy and sorrow; they are usually quiet people, who will not seek advice from one and all as do cerato types, but their indecisiveness makes them unreliable people to deal with. This dithering is a lack of balance that may communicate itself to the physical and make them prone to sea-sickness or air-sickness, as the motion of boat or plane will unsettle them.

29. Star of Bethlehem (*Ornithogalum umbellatum*)

Star of Bethlehem is the remedy for neutralising any shock, mental or physical, and it should be given as quickly as possible after an accident, a fright, or bad news. Shock can of course be delayed, and may manifest itself months after the event. In this case, if the resultant symptoms can definitely be related to earlier shock, then this is the remedy that should be given.

30. Sweet Chestnut (*Castanea sativa*)

Sweet chestnut is for the person who suffers extreme mental anguish, leading to a feeling of hopeless despair. Such people feel that they have reached the absolute limit of their endurance, but they are of strong character and do not commit suicide as a way out. They keep their troubles to themselves, and thus loneliness is added to their absolute despair.

31. Vervain (*Verbena officinalis*)

Vervain is for the tremendously enthusiastic type of

person who forces himself beyond the limits of his physical strength and so suffers strain and tension. Such people hold strong opinions which they try to impose on others. They are the fanatics and the reformers of this world, and in their eagerness they take on too much and overtax themselves.

32. Vine (*Vitis vinifera*)

Vine is for the dominating ambitious type. Vine types are efficient, quick thinking, and certain in their own mind that they are right. They tend to use their gifts to obtain power and to dominate other people. Often there is a cruel streak in their nature and if they obtain power they demand unquestioning obedience from those over whom they have authority. It is the cruel streak that leads to stress and the physical disorders that accompany that condition.

33. Walnut (*Juglans regia*)

Walnut is for those who need to be freed from links with the past, or to be enabled to break habits, so that they may move forwards and realise their very definite ambitions. This type of person is seldom influenced by other people; it is the links with the past or the enslavement to routine which bind them. Walnut will help in any circumstance where a change is contemplated such as moving to a new house, changing one's religion, adopting a new way of life. It is also of help in the natural changes that arise in life such as teething in children, puberty in the teenager, the menopause in later years.

34. Water Violet (*Hottonia palustris*)

Water violet is for the proud aloof type of person. Such people are often talented and sometimes feel superior to others. Although they are gentle and serene by nature, they can be condescending towards others, and at such times may suffer from tension themselves with the resultant physical ailments. Nonetheless they do not interfere with other people and have a deep inner peace.

35. White Chestnut (*Aesculus hippocastanum*)

The white chestnut types are those who have something preying on their minds, so that their thoughts go round and round in circles, getting nowhere. This may even happen when they lie down to sleep. They seem powerless to control these tormenting thoughts, and suffer headaches, insomnia and depression as a result.

36. Wild Oat (*Bromus ramosus*)

Wild oat types suffer from uncertainty which leads to dissatisfaction and ultimately despondency. They are generally talented people, with very distinctive characters, but they seem undecided as to what they want to do. A typical wild oat type will start one career after another, and find satisfaction in none of them. He will then come to feel that life is passing him by and that he is getting nowhere.

37. Wild Rose (*Rosa canina*)

Wild rose is for the type who is apathetic and resigned. It may be due to illness or to a monotonous job in which they are unhappy. This type of person does not complain, but suffers in silence, without seeing that the remedy for his ills lies in his own hands.

38. Willow (*Salix vitellina*)

Willow is for the bitter resentful type, who blames everyone but himself for his troubles. He will say: "What have I done to deserve this?" He will begrudge the success of others. He will be a difficult patient. If anyone tries to help, the willow type will accept it as his due, without any gratitude. The willow types do not realise that it is their own attitude which is responsible for much of their unhappiness.

As well as these thirty-eight remedies, Dr. Bach formulated a composite remedy comprising Star of Bethlehem for shock, Rock Rose for terror and panic, Impatiens for mental stress and tension, Cherry Plum for desperation, and Clematis for feeling of faintness. This he called the "Rescue Remedy". It is used in emergencies to succour and sustain the patient until medical help arrives.

Readers will realise that the above is only a summary of the remedies and their uses. Before attempting self-treatment, they should read Dr. Bach's own books (available from the Dr. Edward Bach Centre, see the Appendix page 149), which give details of how to prescribe.

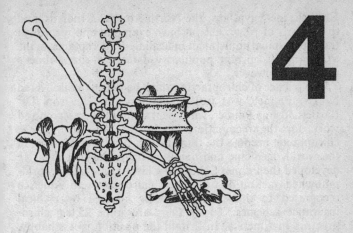

4

CHIROPRACTIC

Chiropractic, sometimes spelt with a final "e", is a system of healing by spinal manipulation. It was discovered, or as chiropractors prefer to put it "re-discovered", by Dr. Daniel David Palmer of Iowa in 1895. The story is that a janitor in the building where Dr. Palmer had his surgery had suffered from deafness for seventeen years, ever since he had bent over and "felt something go" in his back. Dr. Palmer located a painful spot at the exact place the janitor had "felt it go", and when he adjusted the man's vertebra with a quick thrust at this point, the man's hearing was restored. From this simple beginning, the science of chiropractic, as we know it today, was developed.

Spinal manipulation had been known and practised in various parts of the world before this, however. Hippocrates (of Hippocratic oath fame) understood the importance of the back. He advised physicians to "look well to the spine" for the cause of disease. Aesculapius said that complications could result from displacement of spinal vertebrae. The

Chinese, the Egyptians, the North American Indians, and the Maoris of New Zealand have examples and records of the use of spinal adjustment in healing. Its acceptance in the West and its current popularity date from Dr. Palmer's discovery, however.

The science of chiropractic, which had been re-discovered by Dr. Palmer, was further developed by his son, Dr. Bartlett Joshua Palmer, who spent all his life in research and work for the recognition of the art. He lived to see chiropractic become the third largest healing profession in the world, medicine and dentistry being the first two. He developed the Palmer School of Chiropractic into a world-renowned institution, and saw chiropractic in America recognised to the extent of being covered by medical insurance schemes. Today there are some 25,000 chiropractors in America. In Britain the position is less happy. There are only some 200 qualified practitioners in this country.

Chiropractic comes from two Greek words, "cheir" meaning "hand", and "praktikos" meaning "done by". The hands of the chiropractor are in actual contact with the parts of the spine that have to be adjusted. Some people confuse chiropractic with osteopathy. The main difference between the two sciences is one of technique; the philosophy behind them is very much the same. The chiropractor uses what is called a "short lever technique"; the osteopath uses a "long lever technique". This means in a simple form that whereas the chiropractor would hold two adjacent vertebrae in the back and make his adjustment with a quick thrust, an osteopath might hold the shoulder and leg and twist the spine to bring about the adjustment. Sometimes he would use an assistant to help him with this. Another difference between the two sciences is that the chiropractor relies much more on the use of X-rays to see exactly what needs to be done. Indeed, it was the fact that Röntgen discovered X-rays in the same year as Dr. Palmer treated the janitor which enabled chiropractic to develop in the way it did.

There is a philosophical basis to the art. Chiropractors believe that a Universal Intelligence exists, call it "God" or what you will, and that within every human being, there is a part of this intelligence which directs the functions of the body. It is this intelligence which makes us breathe or blink or sneeze, and on a bigger scale makes the body fight disease or heal itself. Illness, they claim, occurs when something interferes with this intelligence.

The chiropractor believes that this intelligence within controls the body through the nervous system. The brain monitors the functions of every organ through nerve pathways. The spinal cord is an extension of the brain, and special nerves leave the spinal cord as it passes down the spinal column, going out to various organs and parts of the body. Thus, there is an intricate system of nerve pathways linked through the spinal cord passing up the spinal column to the brain. Because of this any displacement of the vertebrae, even slight, may compress a nerve channel sufficiently to reduce its normal function, and then the organs which that nerve channel serves will suffer. The chiropractor uses a new term "subluxation" for the condition where the bones of the spinal column are sufficiently displaced to interfere with the correct functioning of a nerve channel.

The spinal column, which is flexible, consists of twenty-four movable segments of bone called "vertebrae", with twenty-three intervening cartilages. In the normal adult, the column has three curves. The first seven vertebrae from the neck to the shoulders form a forward curve and are called cervical vertebrae; the next twelve form a backwards curve and are called dorsal vertebrae; the last five form a forward curve and are called lumbar vertebrae. The spinal column holds the body erect, provides anchorage for the ribs which protect the heart, lungs and other internal organs, absorbs shock through the cartilages, and of course houses the spinal cord. The latter is possibly the most important of its functions.

The chiropractor will study his patient's stance from both front and rear for uprightness of posture, and then from the side for any abnormal variation in the curves, since stance or variation could indicate where the trouble lies. Dr. Palmer stated that there were four degrees of injury to bone structures: fractures, dislocations, subluxations, and misalignments. It is with the last three that the chiropractor is concerned. If he finds dislocation, subluxation or mis-alignment, he must try to discover from his patient's background what has caused it, and by a movement in the opposite direction, he must restore the vertebrae to normal.

Chiropractors do not use drugs. They believe in the inherent power of the human body to heal itself. They prefer not to speak of disease, but to split the word into its two parts "dis-ease", since this gives a truer picture of the state of the patient. They see their task as helping the body to heal itself, and the first step is to take pressure off the trapped nerve that is causing the trouble, by adjusting the spinal column.

A patient's problems may arise originally through accident, as in the case of the janitor whose deafness followed his bending over and feeling something go; they may arise through bad posture or poor working conditions; they may arise through lack of exercise weakening the back muscles; but clearly if the vertebrae are displaced to the extent of compressing a nerve, the resultant disorder may be felt in any part of the body, and not just as simple "backache".

Having first looked for any unnatural stance or restriction of movement in his patient, the chiropractor will test reflexes, rotate joints, and examine tissue tone. Then he will consider the patient's life style. Does he do repetitive work on an assembly line? Does he continually carry heavy sacks of coal? This is the kind of question to be asked. Having established this, he will go on to use special instruments, the neurocalometer and the neurocalograph, to see if there is nerve inflammation. The neurocalometer detects minute heat variations on corresponding sides of the spinal column, and hence indicates where inflammation exists. It is placed at the various points of exit of nerves from the spinal column. Finally, the chiropractor will use X-rays to see what adjustment needs to be made.

Unlike the doctor, the chiropractor will go to great pains to discuss his case with a patient, and will show him the X-ray and explain exactly what has to be done and why. The orthodox medical profession tend to be secretive by comparison, believing it is not good for the patient to know too much. This is true of some patients, of course. There are those who like to know and those who would rather be in ignorance. Naturally, when arranging X-rays, the chiropractor will be aware of the danger of over-exposure, and will take into consideration how recently and how often the patient has been X-rayed.

From his examination, the chiropractor will decide whether he can treat the case or not. (Bone diseases are clearly outside his field and will be referred to an orthodox doctor.) Treatment is not usually painful, and the number of sessions needed will of course be related to how recent or long-standing the disorder is. The first visit to a chiropractor is for examination only. Usually half an hour to an hour is allowed for this consultation. The treatment starts on the second visit. This and subsequent visits will probably take a quarter of an hour.

Basically, the chiropractor would not claim to heal his patient; he would think of his task as enabling the patient's body to heal itself. His job is simply to adjust the spinal column and so relieve the dislocation, subluxation or misalignment.

The training required for such a skilled profession is considerable. There are some fifteen or so colleges in the United States and Canada, and matriculation would be the minimum requirement for entry to a course. In Britain, there is the Anglo-European College of Chiropractic, (for the address see the Appendix page 149). They require three A-level passes in subjects which include Biology or Zoology and Chemistry, for entry to their four-year full-time course.

Subjects studied will be: chiropractic philosophy, chemistry, hygiene, neurology, diagnosis, bacteriology, physiology, X-ray use, the use of the ophthalmoscope, otoscope, sphygmomanometer, stethoscope, percussion hammer, and electro-cardiograph, pathology, dissection, anatomy, psychology, patient's reflexes, tests of injury, and chiropractic techniques. There will be extensive practical work under supervision. At the Palmer College of Chiropractors in the U.S.A., this practical work will occupy 845 hours of the course.

Chiropractic has developed outside orthodox medical

circles and is not officially recognised by the profession, though increasingly many orthodox doctors do recognise the value of the chiropractor's special skills and do refer patients to him. Recognition and registration of the profession would be a safeguard to the public, since without it, anyone can call himself a "chiropractor" with little or no qualification. The main stumbling-block to recognition would appear to be the difficulty of organising clinical trails to test its effectiveness. These are generally conducted by giving one set of patients treatment and another set fake treatments or placebos, using a random selection of cases. This kind of test is easy enough to arrange when the treatment consists of drugs to be assessed, but it is impossible when the treatment under test consists of spinal adjustments.

Chiropractors do not always give dietary advice to their patients, but they do adopt a holistic approach to healing. Orthodox medicine tends to be divided into specialties. Each specialist considers his own limited field; when the patient requires some other treatment, he is sent to another specialist. It is no-one's business to consider the patient's condition as a whole, unless it be his own busy G.P. But the chiropractor would rightly claim that wholeness is nature's intent. Again, orthodox medicine will consider a case cured if they have got rid of the symptoms of which the patient complained and have enabled him to resume his normal way of life. But it is often due to an error in that way of life that caused the patient to become ill in the first place. The chiropractor will see it as his duty to warn the patient what he has been doing wrong.

What conditions can be especially helped by the chiropractor? Very obviously back pain is one answer. About fifty per cent of a chiropractor's patients will go to him in the first place for this problem. Some of these will have been referred by orthodox physicians, since back pain is one of the major causes of lost working hours in Britain, and often there is little that the orthodox doctor can do about it. In serious cases one orthodox treatment is bed-rest with traction. This means stretching the spine with weights hung on the legs, but it does not always produce a permanent cure, and the time the patient has to be in bed (six or seven weeks) lowers muscle tone and makes a recurrence of the original trouble more likely. Chiropractors, using their methods, are likely to have a much better success rate with this kind of trouble.

But neck pain, lumbago, sciatica, arm pains, chest pains, abdominal pains can all be treated by chiropractic. So can many referred pains. Even seemingly unrelated conditions such as asthma, catarrh, indigestion, constipation and menstrual disorders may have their origin in the interference with the nerve channels by subluxation in the spinal column, and then an adjustment may cure what orthodox medicine cannot.

Chiropractic does not pretend to be a cure-all, and chiropractors are trained to recognise those conditions which are outside the scope of their skills. They are ethically bound to refer such patients to other forms of treatment, including orthodox medicine. If you consult a properly trained practitioner and not a charlatan, you should be in safe hands.

How do you find a properly qualified man? The British Chiropractor's Association, (for the address see the Appendix page 149) will send you a register of association members on receipt of a large (9″ x 6″) stamped addressed envelope. Graduates of the colleges in the U.S.A., Canada, or Bournemouth use the title D.C. – Doctor of Chiropractic.

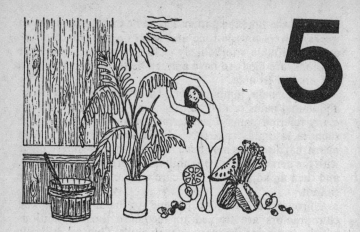

CLINICS AND
HEALTH FARMS, SPAS

Health spas, where people go to "take the waters" are big business on the Continent, where whole towns are geared to exploiting the curative properties of their local mineral springs. Patients normally stay in a hotel, which will provide any special facilities or diets and which will recommend a local doctor. Treatment is hydrotherapy.

The waters can be taken internally by simply drinking them, or they can be used in baths of various kinds. Other treatment such as massage, saunas etc. will be recommended by the doctor, and this will be carried out either in the hotel itself or at a nearby clinic. "Taking the waters" on the Continent is combined with a holiday. The towns are generally in delightful situations, so that sight-seeing can be incorporated; they usually try to arrange a good cultural programme of concerts, theatre, art exhibitions etc.; there are sports facilities. If patients are ill enough to require in-patient treatment, there are sanatoria nearby. Anyone contemplating this kind of holiday with treatment can obtain a list of spas and their special features from the Government Tourist Office of the country concerned. Addresses will be found in the London Telephone Directory.

The chief minerals found in spa waters are: iodine, which is good for high blood pressure, some eye diseases, circulation problems, and some female complaints; iron, which is good for anaemia; sulphur, which is good for rheumatism, skin complaints, and metabolic disorders; sodium sulphate, which is good for gout and obesity and a help in diabetes. Taken internally, the waters correct any imbalance in the body's salts and minerals; taken externally, they tone up the body and improve circulation.

Britain's spas have unfortunately been neglected by comparison with the Continental ones, but facilities are still available in Bath, Buxton, Cheltenham, Droitwich, Harrogate, Llandrindod Wells, Royal Leamington Spa, Strathpeffer and Woodhall. All these spas, both on the Continent and in Britain, are of course linked with traditional orthodox medicine. Doctors recommend them and doctors are in attendance. This does not, of course, lessen their value to those who are seeking healing without harm, as even the most enthusiastic advocate of the alternative therapies cannot find fault with the treatments offered. They are the same as hydrotherapists or naturopaths recommend to their patients.

In contrast to the neglect of spa towns in Britain, health hydros, health farms and clinics for alternative therapy are springing up all over the place. These are run on a somewhat different principle. Patients do not stay at a hotel and combine taking the waters with a holiday. They stay at the hydro or farm or clinic itself, and their whole day is planned for them. It is rather like being an in-patient at a hospital. Patients are told what to do, and in some cases even sent away for failure to conform.

The establishments are usually very comfortable, however, being up to first class hotel standards. Patients will usually stay a week or more. They will be examined either by a doctor or by an alternative practitioner on arrival, and a programme will be drawn up for each individual case. Different centres place the emphasis on different forms of treatment. Some will stress diet; others will be keen on exercise or relaxation techniques. These farms and clinics are not simply places to lose weight, though slimming can be undertaken. They have programmes as well to re-vitalise the system, to de-toxify the body after faulty diet, to tone up the muscles, to overcome the results of stress, and to correct any specific condition of which the patient may be complaining. Usually consultants in naturopathy, hydrotherapy, homoe-opathy, osteopathy, chiropractic, medical herbalism, and acupuncture will be available, some perhaps on the staff, others on a visiting basis. Not only will any curative local waters be used, but also mud baths, exercise, yoga, and diets based on organically grown whole foods.

At many centres, the week will start with a fast, in which the patient will take only lemon tea or fruit juice for the first three days. Colonic irrigation, massage, wax and mud baths, ultra-violet and infra red treatments, underwater massage, saunas, beauty treatments, yoga, and other exercises may all be prescribed. There are often tennis courts, a heated swimming pool, sun terraces, and golf for patients to enjoy.

These places are useful for people who wish to learn what they can do to help themselves, because, of course, although a week at a health clinic might greatly improve a patient's condition, if he went straight back to his old way of life, he would quickly lose any benefits gained. There is an educational element, therefore.

The day is usually fully organised. A typical one might commence with breakfast at 7.30 a.m., then exercises, massage, special treatments and water therapy taking the patient up to lunch-time. After a suitable break for digestion, there might be gymnastics, relaxation, yoga classes, followed by an hour's rest before dinner. If desired, beauty treatments are sometimes fitted into the programme. After dinner there might be some evening activity organised, perhaps games, perhaps a talk or discussion on aspects of health. Smoking and drinking alcohol are often forbidden, but patients do not usually find the régime too spartan, as the places themselves are so comfortable, and they are kept occupied all the time.

There are health hydros, farms and clinics all over Britain, and I have heard good reports of these four: Inglewood Health Hydro, Tyringham Clinic, Champneys in Tring and Champneys in Peebles (for their addresses see the Appendix page 149). For ones in your own area consult the advertisements in 'Here's Health'.

In America, the differences between orthodox and alternative therapies are being bridged in a few holistic clinics, of which some of the better known are Turning Point in Boston, The Clymer Clinic in Pennsylvania, and The Holistic Health Centre in New Jersey.

This chapter on Clinics, Health Farms and Spas would be incomplete without some reference to the new approach to cancer treatment being made in some centres. Dr. Carl Simonton, Director of the Cancer Counselling and Research Centre in Dallas, Texas, believes that gentler non-toxic methods of treatment should be used. Patients' lives should not be unduly lengthened if they are simply going to suffer the pain of treatment in the extra years. The time they have left should be made as meaningful as possible, and then they should be allowed to die. But although cancer is a word like a death sentence to the majority of people it should not be so.

It has been found that a person's emotional life and his personality traits have a definite bearing on the malignancy of the disease. We need to realise that we all have cancer cells in our bodies. In some people they develop; in others they do not. People who bottle up their feeling seem most at risk. Those who can express those feelings and find a release less so. Smokers are at risk. Disturbing emotional experiences can trigger off the development of cancer. Additives to food can exacerbate the situation.

Dr. Simonton believes in counselling patients, and if possible their families as well, since stress within the family can make the patient worse. He tries to get his patients to adopt a positive holistic attitude to life, changing their diet where necessary to avoid those foods which have harmful additives and to incorporate as many fresh organically grown vegetables as they can. He asks them to take exercise, to practise relaxation and meditation, and to try and find a purpose in living. The family, religious advisers, and social workers are all enlisted in the supporting group. The patient will not necessarily get better; certainly there will be no sudden and dramatic improvement, but he will enjoy life more, he will feel that everything possible is being done, and he will meet death more happily.

Some patients in clinics like Dr. Simonton's are asked to use visualisation techniques. They think of the body battling with the cancer cells, using its self-healing mechanism to keep them at bay or even to reduce the tumours. Thus they are given hope and their minds are turned away from the thought of the cancer destroying them. Combined with the other methods of counselling, diet etc., some success is claimed. I have personally met one lady who claimed to have been cured.

It is certainly worth considering whether the present methods of tackling cancer by chemotherapy or radium treatment are the best, despite their successes in some cases. One of these new approaches might yield better results. The body's natural reaction to any situation is to try to heal itself. This reaction is deeper than any conscious thought and is in accord with the self-righting principle of the Universe. What patients need is to give their bodies the best chance for this process to take place, by adopting a wholesome diet, by the avoidance of stress, by a right balance of work, rest and leisure, and by a faith that removes even the fear of death.

Centres of a similar nature to Dr. Simonton's are well-established in Mexico, Germany, Holland, Denmark and the Philippines, and towards the end of 1980, a Cancer Help Centre opened in Bristol. It aims to encourage in patients a hopeful positive attitude of mind and to spread this attitude to their families, so that they can learn how to get well again. Of course it does not claim to cure, but sets out to help the whole person, so that he is more prepared physically, mentally and spiritually to face whatever happens.

As in Dr. Simonton's centre, diet, natural remedies, counselling and relaxation are amongst the techniques used. Patients are encouraged to go for a whole day, when they will be talked to by sympathetic advisers who will seek to uncover any problems or stress. They will be taught how to relax, and how to develop a positive approach to the future whether that future brings life or death. They will be given a suitable midday meal, so that they can see for themselves what their diet is going to be like. They will be helped to plan their future life-style to make the best of the situation. The healing programme of the Bristol centre can safely be used alongside any orthodox medical treatment.

Interested readers should apply to The Cancer Help Centre, (for the address see the Appendix page 150). As it is supported by a charitable trust, donations would be welcomed, but patients' contributions are very modest.

Further information on alternative methods of cancer treatment can be obtained from The Association for New Approaches to Cancer (A.N.A.C.), (for the address see the Appendix page 150). As this again is an entirely voluntary organisation, a self-addressed stamped envelope for reply would be courteous.

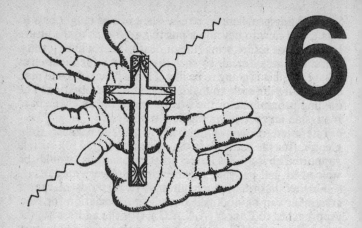

FAITH HEALING

Faith healing is a term not usually used by healers themselves. It is a blanket expression used by the layman to cover those forms of healing, religious-based or otherwise, that depend on contact between a healer and his patient with often no medication or conventional treatment involved. Healers do not generally see themselves as an alternative to orthodox medicine, however, but rather as an aid. Nonetheless, there are many documented cases of their success, where all traditional forms of healing have failed.

There are three main classes of healer. Firstly, there is the religious man, whether clergyman or lay person, who believes that his gift comes from God Himself. He works through the laying on of hands, and through prayer, and traces his tradition back to the earliest disciples of Jesus, who received the power at Pentecost.

Secondly, there is the spiritualist healer. He believes that his work is done under the guidance of the spirits of dead people or of spirits that have never been born into life on this earth. He often works in a trance-like condition. Arigo, the

South American healer, who was known as "the surgeon with a rusty knife" was a healer who came into this category. He was not an educated man, but he performed quite difficult operations without anaesthetic and apparently without pain to the patient, at a speed and with a skill that astonished professional surgeons. He claimed that when doing this he was taken over by the spirit of a German, Dr. Adolphe Fritz, who died in 1918. Dr. Fritz would also dictate prescriptions through Arigo. This class of healer often uses orthodox surgical techniques and drugs, as indeed Arigo did, so that this class of healing does not quite come within the category of this book. However, some of these spiritualist healers go through the motions of performing surgery just above the flesh, without actually touching the patient. They seem to be operating on the psychic body of the patient, and by healing the psychic body they get a corresponding healing of the physical body.

Finally, there is the healer who recognises that a power flows through him to the patient, but rather than think of it as a spiritual or supernatural force, he prefers to believe that it is a natural power, like magnetism or electricity, which some people are able to tap and transmit to others with beneficial effect.

Healing has a long history. The Chinese knew of these methods 5000 years B.C. The Egyptians thought all cures of illness were revealed by the Gods. One of their earliest healers was Imhotep, who lived 2700 B.C. Jesus Christ, whom many believe to have been the Son of God, was the Supreme example of a Divine Healer, but His healing methods were not unknown before His day. The Essenes practised healing, and some people believe that Mary and Joseph, the parents of Jesus, were themselves Essenes, and that they passed on their knowledge to Him. Jesus told his followers that they should practise what he had done, and indeed he said "greater things shall ye do". He clearly believed that healing was within their power. During the first and second centuries after His death, the Church tried to carry on healing, but gradually it split into two conflicting groups. On the one side were the prophets and with them the healers; on the other side were the bishops and priests, the establishment. The latter group gradually became the official Church, and healing died away until it was outlawed.

In the modern Christian Church, it has been recognised from time to time that some people have this gift of healing, but in general the Church tends to think that God works through orthodox medical channels to bring about cures. It is only in sects such as the Pentecostal ones that Divine Healing is practised on any scale. The Christian Scientists have a rather different approach. They believe that all sickness is thought-induced, and that understanding this truth will heal. This is rather different from the kind of healing we are thinking about in this chapter. Christian Scientists are in the tradition of those who practise auto-suggestion.

What is common to all three groups of healers is that they all have a power to affect the patient for good. It has generally been found that the patient does not necessarily have to believe in what the healer is doing for it to work, though it can help if he does. Nor does the healer necessarily have to hold any particular religious belief or to be able to explain what he is doing. It seems that some men can heal and others cannot, though those healers who do not attribute what they are doing to the supernatural, that is the third class, tend to believe that the potential is within every human being. It is simply a question of tapping powers not fully understood at the present time.

Healers in any category do not generally claim any credit for what they are doing. They see themselves as channels through which God or the Spirits or the Power can work. They have been given the gift and they have the duty to use it. Therefore many of them will not accept a fee. Only those whose time becomes fully taken up with healing feel that they have a right to charge, and then only so that they can devote themselves full-time to the work. Of course, there are charlatans as in any other sphere, and it is well to be wary, but there are a lot of genuine people.

Christian healing is usually practised inside a church as part of a Healing Service. The Minister will lay his hands on the patient; the congregation will unite in prayer. The healing that flows is believed to come directly from God

Himself.

Until comparatively recently, Christian healing services were almost always associated with the Pentecostal group of Churches, but recently in both the Catholic and the Protestant Churches, there has arisen what is known as the "Charismatic Movement". St. Paul in the Acts of the Apostles, Chapter 2, verses 1-4, writes: "And when the day of Pentecost was fully come, they were all with one accord in one place. And suddenly there came a sound from heaven as of a rushing mighty wind, and it filled all the house where they were sitting. And there appeared unto them cloven tongues like as of fire, and it sat upon each of them. And they were all filled with the Holy Ghost, and began to speak with other tongues, as the Spirit gave them utterance." The Charismatic Movement is an attempt to recapture this experience, primarily with the idea of making men whole again, and carrying with this the unleashing of the gifts of speaking in tongues and healing which came upon the original disciples at that time.

Christian healers may have the fundamentalist idea of God as a Being in whose image man has been created. Others will think of God as an indefinable Spirit. Jesus said that God was a Spirit and that those who worshipped Him must worship Him in spirit and in truth. These healers will be thinking of God as the motive power for good in the Universe, the self-righting principle that helps the body to heal itself. It is perhaps helpful if we can rid ourselves of the idea of God as an old man in the sky, who works miracles by setting aside natural laws, and think of Him as a Spirit, a Being beyond human definition, but indwelling in all His creation and at the same time transcendent. Jesus taught us that He was a loving God. A loving God is not a Being who needs to be entreated by prayers to set aside the laws He has made. He is the power that is working through those laws for the best. He is continually seeking wholeness in the Universe and whether a particular patient is healed or dies, His will is for the good.

Over the centuries, the Catholic Church has from time to time recorded miracles, performed by God through priests or monks or nuns. Usually after their death such people will be canonised as "saints" after exhaustive enquiries into the genuineness of what they have done. Sometimes these saints have been associated with a particular place, as was Bernadette with Lourdes, and then this will become a place of pilgrimage for the sick. In Lourdes the healing channel is water. Even carrying it away to sick people at home sometimes benefits.

Spiritualist healers have a different approach. Like Christians, they believe in life after death. They also believe that certain people called "mediums" have the power to be contacted by departed spirits. They reason that when a person dies, he will carry on the work he has been doing on earth, but on a different plane. Thus a doctor when he dies would carry on with his study of medicine and with his healing work. Then, like Dr. Fritz, whom Arigo claimed possessed him, the spirit of a departed doctor would use a medium to help earthly patients.

Medicine men in primitive tribes often went into a trance to diagnose what was wrong with a patient. This is what the modern medium does. Since illness in primitive times was often attributed to evil spirits, the medicine man would be called upon to cast them out and make the patient whole. The Church today has a service of exorcism for this situation, but mediums do not only deal with evil spirits.

The third tradition of healing today is not done by priests or spiritualist mediums; it is done by laymen, healers who do not attribute what they are doing either to God or to departed spirits, but who simply believe they are tuning in to natural forces. In this they are not necessarily being irreverent. Most Christians would say that anything that is good comes from God, and hence this natural force which healers are tapping comes from God too.

The commonest technique of all healers in all three categories is the laying on of hands. There are simple examples of the value of this act, even when it is done by someone who is not a healer. A mother will smooth the brow of a fevered child; a sister, looking at a scratched hand, will say "I'll kiss it better"; a friend hearing of disaster will take a hand in his. Such simple acts have a well-known soothing effect, and often physical conditions such as pain or fever will respond. Healers are doing this on a bigger scale or to a higher degree.

Research has been done into what actually happens when a healer lays his hands on the patient. Using encephalographs, which measure rhythms of electrical activity in the brain, it has been found that healers have an unusual brain wave pattern. Maxwell Cade, one of the foremost researchers in the field, calls it "State Five". When he lays on his hands, the healer is able to impose this pattern on the patient's brain waves. They thus become in tune with each other. The patient becomes relaxed and at the same time more alert, and his body is put into the state where it can most readily heal itself. Energy flows from the healer to the patient.

Healers and patients will sometimes say that their hands feel hot or cold, but the phenomenon is not necessarily observed on all occasions. Indeed, it is not actually necessary for the healer to touch his patient. Sometimes just holding his hands near to the patient will be enough.

How does healing work? No-one really knows. It is clear, however, that human beings are more than just physical creatures. We are body, mind and spirit, and the three interact. Jung and Freud have revealed to us the power of the subconscious mind, and what Jung calls the "collective subconscious", wherein is stored experiences of generations. Belief can work wonders. All doctors know the placebo effect, in which patients who are given a pill with no curative qualities whatever will respond in exactly the same way as those who are given genuine medicine, provided they are not told that the pill is useless. It is a curious fact, however, that healing will work independent of the patient's belief in its efficacy.

Apart from the laying on of hands, there is another form of healing that is quite common, that is absent healing. Given a photograph, a lock of hair, a spot of blood, or simply the knowledge that a patient needs help, will enable some healers to concentrate on the case, and healing will be transmitted with no physical contact at all. Distance seems no object. The theory seems to be that power is transmitted through the etheric, in much the same way as happens in radionics.

Group healing is also practised. People interested in healing will form a group to use their power in the service of others. Groups vary in their methods and composition. When they gather under the auspices of a church, they will usually start their meetings with a hymn or a prayer. They will then settle down, relax, and try to think of the purpose of their gathering, before the first patient is brought in. The leader will lay his hands on the patient, and the others may hold out their hands towards him. All will imagine light and power flowing towards the patient. Some groups believe it is helpful for a second patient to arrive a little time before the first leaves, particularly if the second patient is unfamiliar with healing. It adds to his confidence, gives him time to get his bearings, and overcomes any initial anxiety.

If a group is not meeting in a church or other sacred place, the leader will want to cleanse the room physically and spiritually, before the meeting takes place, so that it is filled with light and goodness, and there is no room for evil forces or spirits. He will do this by prayers, and the group will discipline themselves to put away all evil and selfish thoughts. There are powers of darkness as well as of light, and all who deal with these little-understood forces should be aware of the dangers.

Groups practise absent healing in the same way as individual healers. People will write in and ask for help; friends will bring sick relatives to their attention. The group may pray for each one by name, or they may simply hold them in their thoughts and will them to be healed.

Many healers, even those who are not spiritualists, believe that we have an etheric body inside our physical body. This etheric body is the counterpart of our physical body. It will leave the physical body when we die and continue to exist on another plane. Christians would call it the spirit or the soul. Because this etheric body permeates the physical body, sickness of the physical body is reflected in the etheric body and vice versa. So, by healing the etheric body, the physical one can be healed as well. Whether this provides an explanation of why healing works or not is debatable. Certainly in many cases healing does work.

A century ago, doctors were coming to believe that disease was purely physical; it was caused by germs, viruses, and poisons attacking the body. Because the cause was physical, the remedy was physical too. Doctors treated by bleeding, purging, or administering drugs. Medical students in those days were taught that the mind had no part to play. Even mental illness was treated with drugs or with surgical intervention. It is only within the lifetime of the present generation that we have seen a shift in orthodox medical circles to the view that the mind and the emotions have their part to play in sickness and health, and to the belief that the alleviation of stress can be a big step to curing the patient. Even cancer is believed to be related to stress. It is perhaps in this field of overcoming stress that the healer can help most, perhaps by imposing his brainwave patterns on the patient, perhaps by simply instilling confidence and optimism. Very few healers of any category reject other forms of medicine. They see their part as working with doctors, naturopaths etc., not as being in opposition.

Healers will sometimes learn what is wrong with a patient from what he tells them or from his past medical history. However, they have diagnostic methods of their own as well. Some can tell where the trouble lies simply by running their hands over his body, and noting where a reaction is produced. This may well be far away from the expected seat of pain, and may reveal other conditions besides the one complained of. Some healers will use a pendulum in their diagnosis. They will hold it over the patient's body at various points. It reacts in much the same way as the water diviner's dowsing stick. Some healers find that the pendulum oscillates over trouble spots, others that it moves clockwise in a circle, others that it moves anti-clockwise. The behaviour of the pendulum varies with different healers.

We may ask what cases will benefit from faith healing? Spiritualists would say any case, because the spirits are qualified beyond man's abilities. Probably healing is best suited to non-physical causes of illness, but it is unwise to be dogmatic, as thousands of people have been helped even after being given up by their doctors. Even if healing fails and the patient dies, a healer with religious faith would say that this is not failure. Death is not the end, and if it is the patient's time to die, perhaps this is better than to keep him alive. Certainly, in some cases, the prolongation of life by intensive care and life support machines is not the best thing for the patient unless he has some hope of returning to a meaningful existence. The quality of living must always be taken into account.

With the field so open to fake spiritualist mediums, charlatans of one kind and another, it is wise to be careful whom you consult, when you seek healing. The names and addresses given in the Appendix page 150 will provide reliable contacts. The list is not exhaustive. Your clergyman might be able to put you in touch with other sources.

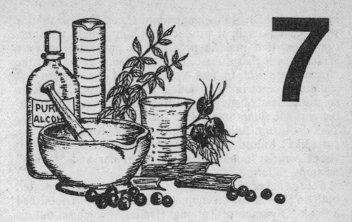

HOMOEOPATHY

Homoeopathy dates back to the end of the 18th century, and to Dr. Samuel Hahnemann of Meissen in Saxony. He was a qualified doctor of medicine, and became well known as a translator of scientific works as well as a writer in his own right. Through his research into the chemistry of drugs, he became friendly with Lavoisier, the great chemist.

The current medical treatments in Dr. Hahnemann's day were those expounded by Dr. Brown of Edinburgh. They were bleeding or sedatives for those who were thought to be over-stimulated, and stimulants for those who were not. Very similar ideas were being taught by Broussais in Paris. He saw all disease as a form of gastro-enteritis, and recommended bleedings and purgings as the cure. Dr. Hahnemann was horrified by these teachings and resolved to look for an alternative remedy.

In 1790, he found one. Quinine had been used by South American tribes to treat malaria, and the practice had spread to Europe. The general belief was that the drug was an antidote. But Dr. Hahnemann found that if he took quinine when he was well, it produced in him exactly the same symptoms that malaria produced in patients who were afflicted with that disease. From this he deduced that the effects were not in fact symptoms of the disease but symptoms of the body's reactions to the disease. If that were so, it was clearly better to assist the body's reaction, that is to increase the symptoms, rather than to try to combat them. This deduction linked up with an age-old idea that "like cures like". Indeed, the world homoeopathy comes from two Greek words "homoios" meaning similar and "pathos" meaning suffering.

For the next twenty years, Dr. Hahnemann experimented both on himself and on volunteers, and in 1810, he published a book "Organum of Rational Healing", which set out his case for the homoeopathic method of treatment. His theories were, meanwhile, being confirmed by Dr. Edward Jenner, who was treating smallpox by vaccination. He was giving a small dose of the disease to stimulate the body's resistance to the main onslaught when it came. This tallied with the homoeopathic theory of like curing like.

During his years of experimentation, Dr. Hahnemann had tried different dosages of the drugs he was using, and he found that to dilute the strength of a drug by shaking it up in water tended to increase its effect rather than to decrease it. He called this dilution "succussion" or "potentising" the drug. Other doctors were scornful. They asked, "How can diluting a drug make it more powerful?" Apothecaries too united against Hahnemann, because their business was going to suffer if less drugs were used. Because it was the custom in those days for doctors to prescribe drugs, and apothecaries to make them up, they found they had grounds to prosecute Dr. Hahnemann for invading their province and dispensing.

A court in Austria forbade him to practise, and he returned to his researches in Leipzig, where he was a lecturer in medicine at the University. He had supporters, however, and when Prince Schwarzenburg wanted to try Hahnemann's treatment, the Emperor could hardly refuse. He ordered that no further action should be taken against

Hahnemann. Schwarzenburg was cured by Hahnemann's homoeopathic methods, even though bleedings and purgings had failed, and though he subsequently had a relapse as a result of returning to his old way of life, Hahnemann's fame was secure.

In 1831, he had a wonderful opportunity to demonstrate the value of his treatments. A cholera epidemic reached Europe from India. Of the patients who were given conventional treatment, 821 died; of those whom Hahnemann treated by homoeopathic medicine, only six died. Hahnemann came to Paris, and his methods soon spread. When he died in 1843, they were widely known.

His book was reprinted five times, and in later editions, Hahnemann changed his thesis slightly and began to enunciate the theory behind homoeopathy. He had earlier said that medicine should help the body's self-healing process. Now, he began to talk of a "vital force" in the body. This vital force could be called "energy" or "consciousness" or the "universal intelligence" of chiropractors, and Hahnemann said that it was this which gave rise to the body's immune system and made the body heal itself. It was the vital force that distinguished a live man from a dead one; it was the "Ch'i" of acupuncture, the "Ki" of shiatzu. Like the acupuncturist, Hahnemann came to see disease as an imbalance in this vital force, and treatment became a question of restoring that balance.

Like all the other alternative therapies, therefore, homoeopathy had a holistic approach. The patient had to be seen as a whole man in his environment, and all factors pertaining to his state, not just his present symptoms, had to be considered when dealing with him. The patient's physical, mental, social, emotional and even spiritual state would affect his health, and the remedy prescribed must be for his whole state of being.

Even in his lifetime many orthodox doctors were impressed with Dr. Hahnemann's work, and today, some doctors in the National Health Service practise homoeopathy in addition to orthodox techniques. There are also lay practitioners, who do not have a medical degree.

The homoeopath's diagnosis tends to involve a lengthy

consultation. He will spend a minimum of an hour with the patient on a first visit, finding out all about him. He will want a complete picture, since the variation of a particular disease which attacks the patient will depend on the kind of person the patient is. To a homoeopath, a cold is not the same thing to one patient as to another.

At the end of the first consultation, a remedy will be prescribed, and the patient will be told to take it for a month or so, in order that its effects can be assessed. Environmental factors and particularly stress have to be considered in the treatment, and on these matters the homoeopath will advise. He may also recommend changes in a patient's diet, though this is less common amongst homoeopathic practitioners.

The homoeopathic remedies are very numerous. They can be of plant, mineral or even animal origin, though plants are probably the commonest source. Sometimes tinctures are made of the whole plant when it is in flower; sometimes only a part, the bark or the leaf or the root is used. They are put into solution in pure alcohol. Some minerals which are insoluble are ground up with lactose granules several times, a process Hahnemann calls "tituration". One part of the remedy is mixed with ninety-nine parts of the dilutant, giving a simple potency. Then one drop of this simple potency will be used with ninety-nine drops of the dilutant to give a second potency. Medicines can be potentised even up to ten thousand times.

When this is done, it will be realised that the quantity of the original substance left is very minute indeed, and to understand how such a trace can do any good at all, we must understand the basis of homoeopathic thought. Homoeopaths believe that once an active substance has been released from its physical manifestations, its spiritual energies are released, and that it is on this level that it will be able to help the patient. It is really the spirit of a substance that is being used.

All homoeopathic drugs have been tested on healthy people, and the results noted, so that when the homoeopath meets with an illness producing certain symptoms, he looks for the drug that will produce those same symptoms in a healthy person. Every tincture used has gone through the process of shaking called succussion, to release in it the vital force needed to heal.

Orthodox medicine believes in getting rid of the particular microbes which cause the illness, but homoeopaths know that doing this often opens the way for other microbes to take over, and in time the original microbes even will develop immunity to the drug being used.

Homoeopaths have to confess that they do not know how their system works; they can only say that it does. In this, they are in very much the same situation as acupuncturists, who cannot point to the meridians of Ch'i because they are not there in a physical sense, but who know that they must have an existence or their healing system would not work.

Because homoeopathy works by stimulating the disease to a minute degree, in order to enable the patient to resist it more strongly, the patient will often get worse before he gets better. The remedy must be given time to assert itself, and this is why he is usually asked to continue taking it for at least a month, before it is changed.

A new development today is the extension of homoeopathy into veterinary practice. Animals seem as responsive to this form of treatment as do humans.

What kind of training do homoeopaths have? A large number of them are fully-trained orthodox doctors of medicine who have taken an additional course in homoeopathy. Since they are qualified to practise either therapy, they will use the treatment that seems best in any particular case. Such doctors use the degree M.F.Hom. as well as their medical degrees, and of course they are forbidden by professional ethics from advertising. They are the only practitioners of the alternative forms of medicine who can be consulted under the National Health Service. Courses for such doctors are run at The Faculty of Homoeopathy (for the address see the Appendix page 150). A register of qualified practitioners is kept.

There are also lay practioners. Part time courses for students without medical qualifications are available at The Society of Homoeopaths (for the address see the Appendix page 150). These are usually of three or four years' duration. Some lay practitioners are entirely self-taught, and must be judged by their results.

Many people try to treat themselves with homoeopathic remedies bought in chemists or health stores. In the case of minor complaints, this is not very different from taking orthodox proprietary medicines, and may be more beneficial than the latter. It is infinitely better to consult a qualified homoeopathic practitioner, however, because when you try to treat yourself, you are back to the practice of treating the complaint rather than treating the patient as a whole man.

What conditions will most benefit from homoeopathy? The answer is almost anything except cases where urgent surgery is imperative. As we have seen, one of Dr. Hahnemann's earliest successes was in the cholera epidemic of 1831. It is perhaps more pertinent to ask what type of patient will most benefit from homoeopathic treatment? There is this spiritual element involved. The traces of the drug after it has been diluted or succussed are so minute that we may readily believe that only the spirit is left, the substance having already gone. This being so, the treatment will clearly appeal more to people who believe that there is more to life than the physical elements. The hard-headed materialist, who scoffs at anything he cannot see, touch, taste or understand, is likely to have less faith in homoeopathy and in any treatment, be it homoeopathic or otherwise, where faith plays some part.

The homoeopath is right in his belief that it is the whole man that counts. Even in severe conditions, the patient's attitude is of great significance. A patient who is frightened or who thinks his case is hopeless will give up the fight; another with exactly the same disease will fight it and make the best of life. Such a patient has a better chance of recovery.

With so many self-taught homoeopaths around, and the limited training of some of the others, who may only have taken a correspondence course for example, it is clearly best to seek treatment under the National Health Service, so that you will see a qualified doctor. A register of those practising homoeopathy can be obtained from The Faculty of Homoeopathy (for the address see the Appendix page 150). You will almost certainly find at least one in any main city.

Failing this, enquiries for a suitable, qualified lay practitioner can be made by sending a stamped addressed envelope to one of the following organisations:

The British Homoeopathic Association, The Hahnemann Society, or The Society of Homoeopaths. (For their addresses see the Appendix page 150.)

These societies only register practitioners who meet their standards in knowledge, practice and ethics. Remember, however, that outside the N.H.S., you will have to pay private fees.

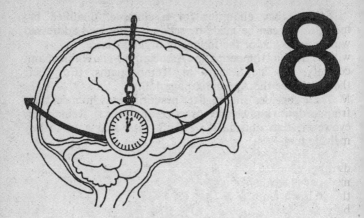

HYPNOTHERAPY

Hypnotism has acquired an unfortunate image today, due to its use as an entertainment in the music halls by stage magicians, and due to a fear that the patient is placing himself too much in the power of the hypnotist. A high degree of trust will be required before a patient will seek treatment from a hypnotherapist, and equally there must be a high degree of responsibility and professional ethics on the part of the practitioner.

The use of hypnotism in healing had its origins in the work of Dr. Franz Mesmer, a Viennese doctor of the 18th century. Mesmer's theory was that the Universe was filled with a magnetic fluid; he considered that illness resulted from an imbalance of this fluid; he believed that the patient could be restored to health by bringing about a right balance of the fluid, using magnetic contact to do so. There are echoes in this theory of both the idea of the etheric, which is met in faith healing and in radionics, and of the balance of yin and yang, which is met in acupuncture.

Mesmer came to Paris and set up a consulting room. The main feature of his treatment was a large oak tub containing water and iron filings. From this tub, called a "baguet", which stood in the centre of the room, protruded rods and cords. Patients would hold these against the affected parts of their body whilst soft music was played to relax them. Mesmer would then make a dramatic entrance, and moving from patient to patient, he would either fix them with his eyes or sometimes touch them with a wand, as if he were a magician.

The majority of his patients were suffering from nervous disorders, and were particularly susceptible to these methods of treatment, but some claimed to be cured of other things, such as asthma, paralysis, and even deafness and blindness. Mesmer himself believed that he was able to heal them by communicating a kind of healing magnetism to them. In time he went on to dispense with the theatrical trappings, as he found that by just staring into their eyes he could establish a rapport and open the way for the healing fluid to flow.

Mesmer's system came to be called mesmerism, after him, but neither Mesmer himself nor any of his contemporaries grasped the idea that the process was a power of the mind. They all thought of it as a force like magnetism that passed between the practitioner and his patient. Mesmer died in 1815, and the Marquis de Puysegur and his brother, the Count Maxime, carried on the practice of mesmerism at their chateau in Buzency, France. It was they who first observed the sleepiness that came over people who were mesmerised, and who saw how easily they were open to suggestions.

In the 1820's, a Portuguese Abbot, the Abbé Faria, who was also experimenting with mesmerism, concluded that there was no such thing as this magnetic fluid that Mesmer had talked about. The Abbé found that he could make his patients go to sleep, simply by telling them to do so. He also discovered that if he sent a person to sleep and then told that person to do something on a given signal when he awoke, the patient would obey the command, even though he was no longer under the Abbé's influence. This phenomenon is now called "post-hypnotic suggestion", though the word hypnotism had not then come into use. Today post-hypnotic suggestion often forms part of a treatment by a hypnotherapist. At the same time, it is one of the features of hypnotism that most awakens a patient's anxiety and makes him reluctant to entrust himself to this form of treatment.

One of the first Englishmen to use mesmerism was John Elliotson. After he had seen a demonstration in France, in 1837, he began to use the technique as an anaesthetic for performing operations. His colleagues were sceptical, but he found that he could perform many operations on patients without causing pain, if he put them into a mesmeric trance first. He also used mesmerism to treat nervous complaints and hysteria.

A Scottish surgeon, John Esdaile, who was working in India, took up this use of mesmerism. He explained the effect in similar terms to Mesmer himself, speaking of a healing fluid that passed from doctor to patient. It was James Braid, another Scotsman, who finally did away with these ideas. He introduced the term "neuro-hypnotism", which soon became shortened to "hypnotism", which is the word we use today.

Hypnotism might have continued to be widely used, but about this time, chloroform and ether were coming into common hospital practice as anaesthetics, and doctors preferred these chemical substances which they could see and understand rather than some mystical power of the mind which they could not explain. Braid had, however, prepared a paper on his work, and he read it in the French Academy in 1860. His reading caught the interest of a French country doctor, Ambrose-Auguste Liébault.

So keen did Liébault become to develop the techniques that he persuaded patients to let him use hypnotism in their treatment by offering to treat them free if they would accept this as an alternative to drugs. His technique of hypnosis was virtually the same as that in use today. He would seat the patient comfortably, or ask him to lie down. He would ask the patient to close his eyes, and then suggest that he was becoming more and more sleepy, until the patient did in fact sink into what was a hypnotic trance. When the patient was in this state, Liébault found that he could suggest a patient's disorders were disappearing and they would disappear.

Liébault worked in obscurity in Nancy for twenty years. He brought out a book on his cases in 1866, but it failed to sell. His chance of recognition came in 1882. During that year, Professor Hippolyte Bernheim went to Nancy to expose him. Liébault had cured a patient with whom Bernheim had had no success, and Bernheim simply could not believe it. However, what he saw in Nancy made such an impression on him that he became a pupil and ardent supporter of Liébault.

Some years later, Sigmund Freud, who had gone to France to study under the neurologist Charcot, also went to Nancy and was impressed with Liébault's work. Charcot was teaching that hypnosis was an abnormal state always associated with hysteria, and he brought back Mesmer's idea of a magnetic influence, but Liébault and Bernheim were showing that any patients, and not just hysterical ones, could be open to hypnotic suggestion.

Freud's use of hypnosis was to enable his patients to recall and discuss incidents they had forgotten with their conscious minds. By bringing these incidents into the open and coming to terms with them, they could be helped towards a cure. Later, Freud discarded hypnosis as a means of doing this, and favoured the "free association of ideas" method. In this, the psychologist encourages a completely conscious patient to talk about whatever comes into his head. This method is sometimes used in psycho-analysis.

A misconception about hypnosis is that the patient cannot be told to do something when in a trance which he would refuse to do in his normal state. If this were true, some of the apprehension about hypnotism would disappear, but unfortunately modern experiments have indicated otherwise. We still do not know exactly how hypnotism works, but we do know that some surprising cures have resulted from its use.

A modern hypnotist will use a technique very like Liébault's. He will make sure that the patient is comfortable and relaxed in a warm room. He may use a mirror or some object like a watch swinging on a chain to focus the patient's attention and to induce physical tiredness of the eyes. He may, on the other hand, rely purely on suggestion, repeated quietly and monotonously, until the patient lapses into trance. If the patient is nervous, it is unlikely that the suggestion will go as far as trance during the first session. The hypnotherapist will simply try to build up confidence. If the patient can simply relax and talk, this will be helpful, and will build up confidence for a future session.

Hypnotherapy today is practised by some doctors as part of their general medical care. It is also practised by hypnotherapists who may have no medical qualifications. Even stage hypnotists have been credited with cures, however, so the absence of a medical degree does not necessarily condemn a therapist.

There are two main uses of hypnosis today. The first is to put the patient into a trance so that he will reveal emotional problems that are troubling his subconscious mind. This is the use Freud made of it. The psycho-analyst is more likely to use free association of ideas to achieve the same effect without hypnosis. The second use is to make post-hypnotic suggestions. This use can even get rid of symptoms, but the danger of that is that whilst symptoms can be got rid of, the underlying condition to which they were a guide may still be there, and then the hypnotist has simply turned off the warning lights. His patient might be better off with his symptoms, since they would point the way to correct treatment along orthodox lines.

Post-hypnotic suggestion needs especial care. A case is recorded of a stage hypnotist who suggested that his patient would fall asleep every time he hummed a certain tune. This worked all right on stage, to the audience's delight, but later the patient responded in the same way whilst driving his car, simply because he chanced to hear the tune on his car radio. Fortunately, others were in the car, and disaster was averted, but further hypnosis was required to restore the man's functions to normal.

Hypnosis can still be used as an anaesthetic, but patients do not generally like it. Most people do not want to see or know what is being done to them by a surgeon. Many are afraid that it may not work, and that they will wake up in the middle of an operation to unendurable pain. The only use made of hypnosis as an anaesthetic in Britain today is in the case of childbirth. However, in the United States, dentists sometimes use it. The curious thing in this case is that not only is pain conquered but there is no bleeding either.

The main conditions that can be helped by hypnotherapy are mental conditions such as stress, hysteria and anxiety. Some physical disorders such as asthma and insomnia respond. Excellent results have been obtained in helping patients to overcome addictions, such as smoking, excess use of alcohol, or drugs. People with weight problems have been enabled to stick to their diets.

Treatment depends, however, on a deep measure of trust between patient and therapist. It is wise to select a practitioner with great care, and you are unlikely to be helped by anyone unless you have complete confidence in him.

There is another therapy related to hypnotherapy which can be practised by the patient himself. This is auto-suggestion. It is based on the ideas of Coué. He had his patients say to themselves every day: "Every day and in every way, I am getting better and better". Try it, and believe it, and you will. The value of this kind of positive thinking has been admirably expounded by Dr. Norman Vincent Peale in his book "The Power of Positive Thinking". Thoughts have power to re-vitalise and heal, if we will but use them.

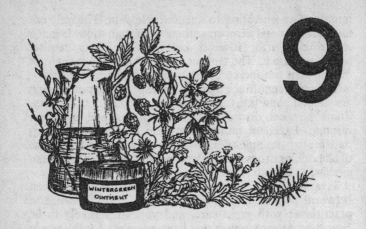

MEDICAL HERBALISM

Plants and herbs have been used to treat illness from earliest times. Even today, animals know which plants are good for them. A household cat will go and eat grass when it is upset. It will also fast. Free-roaming farm animals will move to fresh pastures of their own accord in order to find food containing any trace elements in which they know they are deficient.

At one time in our development, man probably possessed this intuitive knowledge as well, and could treat himself, but as he came to rely more on his intellect and less on his instinct, this knowledge died away. It now only survives in fragments that have been handed down as memories from generation to generation. It is known that the Chinese were practising herbal medicine from at least 3000 B.C. Shen Ming, who reigned at that time, is considered the father of Chinese herbalism. He mixed three hundred and sixty-five different potions for different ailments, corresponding with the number of days in the year. By 1593 A.D. the number of prescriptions had vastly increased, and Dr. Li Shi Chen's pharmacopia, published in that year, contains ten thousand prescriptions. The Greeks, Dioscorides and Galen used herbs in their treatment.

Later herbalists had to test by trial and error those things which had not been remembered and handed down. Country communities in various parts of the world would, however, have their "wise woman" who would be the storehouse of herbal knowledge, and who would dispense prescriptions. Up to five hundred years ago, herbalism was the main traditional medicine.

In the sixteenth century, a Swiss-German doctor, Paracelsus, introduced various inorganic substances into treatment, and though he continued to use herbs as well, this was the beginning of modern drug therapy. The apothecaries and later the big drug houses had a vested interest in seeing that the use of these substances became popular. Gradually, herbalism came to be equated with folklore and old wives' tales, and to be considered amateurish and even unscientific.

Nicolas Culpepper, who lived from 1616 to 1654, wrote a famous "Herbal", which became a household word in his day, and ran through edition after edition. It is still in print today. Unfortunately his book did little to commend herbalism to orthodox physicians, because he was keen on astrology, and as well as giving factual information in his book about where to find the herbs, how to recognise them and how to use them, he included such information as the sign of the zodiac under whose dominion they came. Of one, he says "Jupiter owns this herb"; of another "It is under the dominion of Mars".

When the Industrial Revolution brought hordes of country people into the great cities of Britain, they brought their desire for herbal remedies with them, and as they were no longer able to go out and gather the plants in field or hedgerow, herb shops sprang up to supply them. Doctors, on the other hand, were beginning to isolate the essential elements in plants, and chemists were succeeding in producing those elements synthetically, so that the trend towards a drug-based therapy was growing.

Various attempts were made to protect the interests of

herbalists legally and to give them status, but the first real step forward in this direction was the establishment in 1864 of The National Association of Medical Herbalists. This association received support from the growing interest in herbalism in the United States. The position in that country was somewhat different from that in Britain. In many of the frontier towns, there was no doctor and herbal remedies were the only ones available. The native Red Indians relied on herbs and contributed their own special knowledge of what was efficacious. The basic aims of these early herbalists was first to rid the body of poisons and secondly to stimulate the circulation, but new uses of herbs were constantly being explored.

Although reading a Herbal may give the impression that herbalism simply follows the orthodox medical custom of prescribing a particular remedy for a particular complaint, the approach is different. Herbal treatment is holistic. A qualified herbalist will consider the case history of his patient, his allergies, his diet, any stress he is under. He will take blood pressure, pulse and urine samples. He will look out for deficiencies, which will show up in the eyes or the nails. He will seek to restore balance in the patient, and experiment until he finds the right herb and the right dose. He believes that the patient's body can help itself; he has only got to aid that process.

The trained herbalist today may also be skilled in one or more of the other alternative therapies, such as naturopathy, osteopathy or acupuncture. Like practitioners in these arts, he is concerned not so much with what the patient complains about, but with how he came to be in that condition. If healing is to be permanent, it is always this underlying cause that has to be sought out and put right.

When Asians came to Britain in considerable numbers after the last war, they brought their own special brand of herbalists with them. These were Hakims or wise men. They practised the Unani system of herbal medicine, which came from India and Pakistan. These hakims not only practise amongst the Asian communities in Britain; they will also treat anyone else who chooses to consult them as well, so that a word about their system is not out of place.

Briefly, the Unani School has its historical roots in the Greek teachings of Hippocrates, and the school he established on the Island of Cos in 400 B.C. Like acupuncture, the Unani school uses pulse diagnosis, but the hakim does not claim to feel twelve pulses with twenty-seven qualities in each as does the acupuncturist; the hakim recognises only four qualities: saffra, hot and dry; khun, hot and wet; suda, cold and dry; and bacram, cold and wet. He classifies the remedies in the same way, and the one he will choose in any case, is the one that will counteract the patient's condition. For example, diabetes is considered a cold and wet condition, bacram; therefore, it is treated with a hot dry herb, turmeric.

The herbs most frequently used by the hakim are turmeric, cardamon, thyme, pepper, garlic and mint. He knows many others, of course, but rarely uses more than a few. His approach to treatment like that of his Western counterpart is holistic.

Hakims train at the Unani Medical Colleges in India or Pakistan, and those who obtain qualifications there are classified as Grade A. There are, however, others who train by apprenticeship to a qualified man, and these are classified as Grade B. Some claiming to be hakims in Britain have neither qualification, but are self-taught or even charlatans. If seeking treatment, therefore, it is wise to find a qualified one by consulting the register kept by The Association of Unani and Ayurvedic Practitioners (for the address see the Appendix page 151).

Before the advent of the National Health Service in Britain, doctors' bills had to be paid, and many families would treat themselves for any but the more serious conditions. In those days the "Heath and Heather" catalogue was to be found in most working class homes. This was a commercial catalogue, but it gave the herbal remedies for most conditions, and fulfilled the function of herbalist to thousands of people.

Of those who still prefer herbal remedies today, it is probably true to say that the majority will treat themselves. There are excellent books available, giving descriptions of the plants to be used, where to find them, and how to prepare remedies from them. One such book will be mentioned later on. As examples of what can be done, however, we are going to look at twelve plants, well-known and easily found, which have proven value. This does not claim to be anything more than a representative sample; there are literally hundreds of others.

1. Blackberry (*Rubus fructicosus*)

The blackberry bush grows in hedgerows and woodlands and is sometimes found also on moorland. It has green berries, which turn red and then black when ripe. It is rich in medicinal value. The fruit can be eaten raw or cooked, and is a gentle laxative. A brew of the leaves sweetened with honey is a cure for skin and blood disorders. The same brew applied externally is a cure for eczema. One ounce of the bruised root boiled in water is said to be useful in cases of whooping cough.

2. Broom (*Cytisus scoparius*)

Broom has a yellow flower, not unlike gorse, except that the plant is not prickly. It is found on heathland. A concoction is made from it by taking one ounce of dried tips of the flowering branches and brewing in one pint of boiling water. This is useful against worms, jaundice, dropsy, kidney and bladder troubles. The dose is one tablespoonful morning and night. Great care should be taken to choose true broom, however, as the Spanish broom (*Spartium juncium*) is poisonous.

3. Coltsfoot (*Tussilago farfara*)

This is found on banks and on waste land in early Spring. The flowers are bright yellow. Make a brew consisting of one ounce of the dried leaves to a quart of water, boiling down to one pint. Allow to steep overnight, when the herbs will settle to the bottom and the liquid can be strained off. The medicine is good for coughs and colds, one teaspoonful with honey every three hours. It can also be applied as a hot poultice on the chest. Make freshly as often as required, as a brew will only keep for about three days. Some authorities say that the dried and powdered leaves of this plant can be used as snuff to relieve sinus trouble.

4. Comfrey (*Symphytum officionale*)

This is found in damp places, such as ditches and river banks. It has rough oval leaves, and bluish-pink bell-like flowers. It is a member of the borage family, all of which are highly valued in folk medicine. The leaves are applied externally as fomentations for sprains, swellings, bruises, boils and abscesses. The leaves can also be eaten raw in salads. An infusion can be made with one ounce of leaves in one pint of boiling water, and this is helpful in cases of tuberculosis and other lung troubles. Indeed, in one form or another, comfrey is helpful for almost all ills.

5. Cowslip (*Primula veris*)

The cowslip is found in meadows or on slopes. It prefers chalky soil. It has bright yellow flowers. A few flower heads can be eaten daily with salads. A syrup can be made from the flowers, using one pound of them to one and a half pints of boiling water, and simmering with sugar until a fine yellow juice is obtained. This is taken with water. The herb in its various medicinal forms is good for the nerves and for insomnia or restlessness.

6. Dandelion (*Taraxacum officionalis*)

The dandelion is found on open land, in meadows, and along embankments. It has bright yellow daisy-like flowers. The stems when squeezed exude a white juice. This juice can be applied to warts, blisters, and long-standing sores with good effect. The green leaves can be chopped up and used in salads, when they will have a blood-cleansing effect. The roasted roots are used to make dandelion coffee. This stimulates the kidneys and the liver.

7. Elder (*Sambucus nigra*)

Elder is a shrub that grows in hedgerows, has white flowers and black berries when they ripen. All parts of the plant can be used for some purpose, which makes it a great favourite with country people. The flowers are dried and made into elder tea, a useful remedy for coughs and colds. The berries are made into elder wine, sweetened with honey, and taken as a remedy for sore throats and coughs. The wine is also a laxative. The leaves are made into a brew applied to ringworm, eczema and itching. The inner bark from old branches is powdered and used at the onset of epileptic fits.

The root is made into a brew that is effective in cases of dropsy and kidney ailments.

8. Fennel (*Foeniculum officionale*)

Fennel is found on dry banks, and especially in coastal regions. The flowers are greenish-yellow. The plant has a scent of hay. The leaves are made into an infusion used for gastric ailments, fever, cramp, rheumatism, and diabetes. Externally, they can be applied as a poultice. The hearts of the shoots are used as a laxative. The crushed seeds can be used to make tea, which expels poisons from the system. For this reason it is used against animal bites. The tea is also said to reduce obesity.

9. Golden Rod (*Solidago virgaurea*)

Golden rod is found on open spaces. The flowers grow in tall rods with tiny golden clusters powdered with pollen. An infusion of them is used for digestive ailments. Cases are on record of it being effective in enabling stones in the bladder to be passed. Externally it is used to staunch bleeding. The North American Indians used it for this purpose, and would apply it after battle.

10. Hawthorn (*Crataegus oxyacanthoides*)

Hawthorn is found in hedgerows and woodlands. The small white flowers grow in clusters. The fruits which are small and red are known as "haws". Country children call the leaves "bread and cheese" and will eat them raw. They will also eat the berries at a certain stage of ripeness when they are mushy. The pulped leaves and fruit are used as a poultice for drawing out embedded thorns and splinters, or for whitlows. The flowers and the fruit are a diuretic and also help with sore throats. The berries can be made into a liqueur with brandy. The buds can be added to salad dishes as a tonic.

11. Marsh Mallow (*Althea officionalis*)

Marsh mallow is found on waste land and particularly near the sea shore. The flowers are mauve, and the whole plant is medicinal. The young leaves can be added to a salad and they will stimulate the kidneys. A lotion of the leaves and the flowers can be used as a poultice or to bathe styes on the eyes. A decoction can be made of the root, by adding one quarter pound of the dried root to five pints of boiling water, boiling down to three pints. This helps in urinary disorders, or can be applied externally for sprains, bruises, and muscular aches generally. Boiled in milk or wine, the marsh mallow is a popular remedy for coughs and for bronchitis.

12. Primrose (*Primula vulgaris*)

The primrose is found in woodlands and on banks by streams. It has single pale yellow flowers, and is a favourite with English gypsies as a herbal cure. It is used for over-acidity, high blood pressure, rheumatism, arthritis, and sciatica. The flowers can be eaten raw, and are most palatable if shredded and mixed with honey. The leaves can be added to a salad. A tincture can be made of the whole plant, using ten ounces of plant to one pint of alcohol. The dose is then one to ten drops for insomnia or general restlessness.

If this brief look at what can be done has roused your interest in self treatment, an excellent book to consult is "A Modern Herbal" by Mrs. M. Grieve, published by Penguin Books. This is a veritable cornucopia of remedies.

It is best not to gather herbs by the side of the road or in farmers' fields, where they may have been contaminated by sprays, but to gather them on truly waste ground. Better still, grow your own, or buy ones which have been organically grown. Buying is probably the most practical method for most people, as the time taken to find wild ones in sufficient quantity is considerable, even if you have the botanical knowledge needed to avoid dangerous mistakes. Most of the herbs sold in herb shops are imported from Eastern Europe in these days, and they are organically grown, so are free from any trace of sprays or pesticides.

Herbs are of course a food, which is why so many of them can simply be added to salads or used in cooking. Their health-giving properties are in no way diminished when they are taken in this way. Herbalists will, however, normally make up herbs into infusions, decoctions, tinctures and tablets.

An infusion is made by pouring boiling water or other fluid on herbs or ingredients. A decoction is made by actually boiling the herbs in the water. A tincture is made by soaking the herbs in alcohol.

There are two hundred and fifty plants that can legally be

used as medicines in Britain. There are probably many more that have a therapeutic value.

The time to consult a herbalist as opposed to prescribing for yourself is when you are not quite sure what is wrong with you. Bear in mind that the man who keeps your local herb shop may not be a herbalist. He may simply be a man who sells herbs, knowledgeable as far as which herb will help which condition, but not qualified to diagnose or prescribe. A true herbalist will not just sell you something over the counter. He will want to have a consultation as thorough as any other alternative practitioner, so that he can prescribe exactly what is needed in your particular case.

A complete list of qualified practitioners can be obtained from The National Institute of Herbal Medicine (for the address see the Appendix page 151). This body also runs a full-time four-year training course, and shorter correspondence courses.

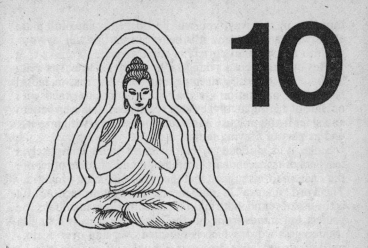

MEDITATION

Meditation is as old as religious belief, and its main therapeutic value is in combating stress. Its religious significance is beyond the scope of this book, but it has formed part of the discipline of hermits, monks, priests, and lay people of many faiths.

Transcendental meditation became one of the "in" things in the 1960's, when the Beatles took it up, and probably this is the form of meditation most familiar to lay people today. Many have been put off, however, by the yellow-robed shaven figures who teach meditation in some of our big cities. But you do not have to go to a guru or teacher to practise meditation, nor do you necessarily have to join a group or a new faith.

The principle behind meditation is that you relax, and empty your mind of those thoughts that chase each other round and round, those worries, anxieties, fears and even hopes that will not let you alone. When you have stilled your thoughts in this way, you will be led gently into full and effective relaxation, and it is believed that this will lay you open to the spiritual powers of the Universe.

This openness has its dangers, however, since evil as well as good can come into an empty mind. For this reason, most teachers of meditation ask their students not to practise it outside of a group until they are experienced. It is even better and safer if you practise it in a religious setting, with prayer, and as part of a living faith.

Since it is difficult to empty one's mind completely, teachers of transcendental meditation and of some other of the Eastern forms suggest that their students chant a mantra. The word "mantra" literally means "thought protection". It is the use of sound, both audible and sometimes inaudible, to protect our minds from our thoughts. It is usually a single meaningless word, which is repeated over and over again, until it drives all extraneous thoughts from our mind. Followers of Hari Krishna, for example, will chant his name repeatedly. Other teachers will give their pupils a letter of the Sanskrit alphabet, whose mere sound is said to transcend language and to put the person who chants it in touch with Universal vibrations.

This in turn, is said to awaken dormant sections of the brain, with beneficial effects, both physiologically and psychologically. An experiment was tried in India, in which young thugs were given the choice between spending a term in prison or studying Sanskrit for one year. Of those who chose to learn Sanskrit, many were transformed into good citizens. Teachers would claim that it was the mere speaking of the sound, putting them in touch with the basic sound of the Universe, that wrought the transformation.

The belief behind mantra-chanting is that sound is the basis of the Universe, and that sound itself creates all forms. If you scatter iron filings on a taut drum, and then play a sound, the sound waves and vibration of the drum will cause the filings to assume a geometrical pattern. This leads to the belief that it is sound that decides the variety of expressions that energy assumes, if we take the modern scientific theory that everything is basically energy. The thought is in St. John's Gospel: "In the beginning was the Word, and the

Word was with God, and the Word was God." It is also found in the Hindu Scriptures, The Vedas: "In the beginning was the Brahma, with whom was the Word." Mantra teachers believe that the "word" thus spoken of, is in each case the primal sound. All the sounds of the world, of the planets, of the spheres, of the universe combine to make this primal sound, and this vibration which gives life is God. Therefore, chanting mantra can put you in touch with God, from whom all healing flows, and men will be healed, since sickness is just being out of tune with the Universe or with God. We have already met this kind of thought in acupuncture, faith healing and other therapies.

But emptying one's mind of thought can be done in other ways besides chanting mantra. You can clear away unwanted thoughts and anxieties by replacing them with a calm, relaxing scene. To make the mind completely empty of everything is difficult, and conscious effort to do so may cause tensions which defeat the purpose. But to fill your thoughts with something pleasant, such as a happy day you spent at the seaside or in the country will have the same effect as chanting a mantra. It will displace all the other thoughts. Once you have done that, you have only to relax, and gradually even the pleasant picture you built up will fade away, and your mind will be truly emptied.

Meditation in religion is usually centred on God, or on His will, or on some specific aspect of faith. The emptying of the mind of every selfish earthly and extraneous thought is part of the discipline that turns the believer's attention to the source of his being, the Creator, God. It opens the believer to new understanding, to strength and to peace. As the Psalms say: "They that wait on the Lord shall renew their strength". Another advice in the Bible is: "Be still and know that I am God".

An experience like this is found in the meetings for worship of the Religious Society of Friends, the Quakers, and they call it "centring down". They sit in silent waiting, trying to silence their own distracting thoughts, as well as avoiding the distractions of hymn singing or a preacher, and believing that in this silence, God can speak to them. He may speak inwardly to an individual soul, or He may through His spirit guide one of them into addressing the meeting. The experience of this kind of worship is very like the tuning into the vibrations of the Universe that mantra chanters are seeking. However, since it is done in a Christian setting, the dangers of getting in touch with wrong vibrations are minimized.

The mental relaxation that leads to the state of true meditation is helped by physical relaxation. This too has a beneficial effect on the body. Physical relaxation is best achieved by tensing each muscle in turn, so that you will know what it feels like when tense, and then slowly relaxing it. Try clenching your fist. The muscles of your hand and arm become firm. Slowly unfold your fist. The muscles relax. You can do the same thing with your arm, flexing your biceps, and then letting the arm hang loosely by your side. You can do it with your legs and feet. You can try to pull your stomach in, to tighten the abdominal muscles, and then let them relax again. By taking a deep breath and holding it, you can tense up your chest muscles, and then slowly expel the air to relax them. All your muscles can be tensed and relaxed in the same way, your shoulders, your neck, your facial muscles.

Do these exercises in a quiet room where you will not be disturbed. Have subdued light or no light at all, and lie flat on a comfortable bed or couch, whilst you are attaining this state of complete physical relaxation. The effect of relaxation and meditation is to lower your oxygen consumption and your heart and metabolic rates. This reduces blood pressure, irritability, nervousness and depression. All aggressive feelings will go away. For patients on such drugs as valium, these techniques could enable the dose to be reduced and in time there is a hope that you will be able to do without it altogether.

The causes of stress in our present society are many. City life with its pollution of air and environment, its vandalism, noise, bright lights, its high-rise dwellings, overcrowding, muggings, burglary, traffic dangers, the speed at which everything goes including life itself, the lack of a supportive community, all these are stress-producing factors. But country life, too, has its drawbacks. Loneliness, isolation, and a sense of deprivation may be felt, particularly by the young, who compare their lot unfavourably with city dwellers who have amusements to hand, more stylish shops, and access to sports, culture and wider job opportunities. Work is one of the prime causes of stress. There is the struggle for promotion, the disappointment of being passed by, the fear of unemployment, working with incompatible colleagues or supervisors, the lack of fulfilment in repetitive and seemingly meaningless tasks, the failure to achieve any job satisfaction, or, at the other end of the scale, responsibilities greater than the capacity of the one who has to bear them. Housewives are under stress. If they have all the latest labour-saving devices, they may become bored in the home. If they are struggling with old fashioned equipment, they may feel they are hard done by in comparison with their neighbours, who have these devices. If they take a job to ease the money situation or because of boredom, they may then become over-burdened, and resentful if their husband does not take his full share of household tasks to help. Marriage generally produces stress, particularly if there is fear or suspicion of unfaithfulness, or if it has been entered into when immature, or if love has somehow gone with the passing years. Sex life can produce stress, if there is a divergence in partners' needs or capabilities. Financial problems, discrimination on grounds of race, religion, sex or colour, all cause stress.

Almost all illnesses are aggravated by stress, and people who are subjected to it become more accident prone. They may seek escape in drugs or alcohol and become addicted to one of these. They may find that their stress triggers off allergies. Heart attacks, strokes, ulcers, backache, migraine, constipation, diarrhoea, indigestion are all conditions that can arise from stress. Perhaps even worse is impotence in the male, since worry over his lost ability and its effect on his partner creates even more stress.

Two compensations frequently resorted to are over-eating and smoking. The first leads to obesity; the second can lead to lung cancer.

Any technique that can reduce stress is therefore worth looking into. Meditation is a gentle and harmless one.

Meditation is one of the aspects of yoga, and the physical exercises of yoga are also beneficial to health, as they keep the body supple. Yoga is not everyone's choice of exercise, however, as some of the postures look very difficult to get into, though of course the student will be led gradually by a good teacher from the easy ones into the more advanced. Some Christian people do not like the links with Eastern religions, however, and would prefer to see meditation practised within the framework of their own beliefs.

Whether you take up meditation as part of a religious discipline, or by mantra-chanting, the value of starting in a group rather than alone is that you can be given help with the practical techniques, and the supportive friendship of the group will in itself help to alleviate stress. As well as teachers who advertise, clergymen might well be able to advise where to start. Meditation needs no drugs or external appliances, yet it is undoubtedly effective in its healing processes.

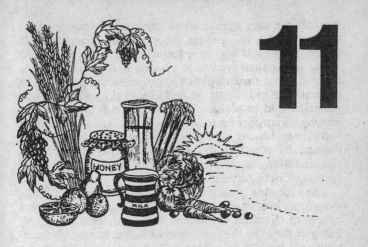

NATUROPATHY AND
HYDROTHERAPY

Naturopathy or Nature Cure, as it is more commonly called, is one of the more revolutionary of the alternative therapies, in that it rejects the whole basis of orthodox medicine, declaring that many of the orthodox treatments do more harm than good, because they are based on a false understanding. According to naturopaths, orthodox medicine has tried and discarded one form of treatment after another, over the centuries, until they enthusiastically settled for Pasteur's germ theory of disease. Now, doctors put all their faith in attacking invading germs with drugs and in surgery where this is not effective.

Yet, say naturopaths, the body is always full of germs and bacteria. They break down dead organic matter into its constituents so that it can be eliminated. Naturopaths see germs, therefore, not as causes of disease, but as Nature's scavengers, ridding the body of disease. They do not deny that disease may sometimes be contracted through germs transmitted to the patient from outside, but this only happens to people who have accumulated toxins and bodily refuse within their systems to provide soil for the disease to flourish. To the naturopath, the cause of disease is always a lowered vitality, due to the body being clogged with waste materials and impurities. This condition is due to wrong feeding, improper care of the body, and bad habits. Hereditary factors also play their part, of course, but a disease, by whatever name it is called and whatever its manifestation, is always caused by these fundamental factors of wrong living.

The orthodox practitioner mainly tries to get rid of the symptoms in his treatment. The naturopath has a different approach. He does not bother very much with symptoms, but gets down to the fundamental causes instead. Naturopaths are fond of describing orthodox cures as merely the suppression of the symptoms. Disease to them is Nature's attempt at self-healing, and the process should be helped, not suppressed by drugs, since to do that is to thwart Nature's work.

Nature cure has been known since antiquity, but the first men in Europe to practise these natural methods of healing were Vincenz Priessnitz, who set up a clinic in Germany, and Johannes Schroth, who did the same in Austria, about the middle of the last century. They were followed by Sebastian Kneipp, Arnold Rikti, Lehman, and Kuhne. In America, Drs. Troll, Kellogg, Lindbahr, and Tilden, who were orthodox practitioners of medicine to begin with, turned to Nature Cure. In Britain, Mr. Stanley Lief was the chief exponent of the system, in the 1920's, and others have followed since, one of the foremost being Harry Benjamin, whose famous book "Better Sight Without Glasses" extended Nature Cure methods to the treatment of eye conditions.

The object of naturopathy is to encourage the body to work efficiently and harmoniously. It considers that to be well is the natural state to which the body will strive, and that there is a built-in self-correcting force, which will bring the body back to health at any time, providing obstacles are removed. These obstacles may be physical. Drug therapies may have contaminated the system. Foods made impure with additives or preservatives, or containing trace poisons as a result of the original crops having been sprayed with chemicals or forced with unnatural fertilisers, may have contributed to this contamination. Bad habits, such as smoking, taking alcohol, not getting enough exercise may have damaged the body mechanisms. Poor posture or stress may have lowered vitality. It is from this way of living and its effects that Nature Cure would save us.

There are three fundamental principles in effecting a cure:

1. The first principle is that all forms of disease are due to the same cause. This is the accumulation of waste material in the body, as the result of wrong living habits, faulty diet, worry, overwork, excesses of any kind and neglect. From this principle, it follows that disease can only be cured by throwing off or eliminating these waste products. In the healthy person, they are eliminated through the bowels, the skin, the lungs and the kidneys, before they can accumulate sufficiently to cause problems, but if a person does not take proper care to remain healthy, the clogging up of the system by these products results in ill-health.

2. The second principle is that the body is always trying to heal itself. Diseases are classified as being acute or chronic. Acute diseases are the early manifestations that all is not well, such as fever, colds, diarrhoea, or skin eruptions. These are all the body's attempts to throw off accumulations of waste material. If these attempts are suppressed by drugs, as is the practice in orthodox medical treatments, the naturopath says that chronic diseases will follow. The misguided attempt to cure the acute condition forces the waste products, which might otherwise have been thrown off, deeper into the system, and the result is a chronic condition. The form this takes will depend on the bodily condition and the hereditary tendencies of the particular patient, but naturopaths claim that all chronic diseases arise in the first place through wrong medical treatment of acute diseases. It is a sweeping and revolutionary doctrine.

3. The third principle is that the body does have the power

to restore itself to health, providing it is allowed to do so. The cure lies not in surgery nor in drugs, but in the self-righting power of the human system. The aim of Nature Cure is always to give the body the best conditions in which this self-righting principle can operate.

In a simple form, we can see this self-righting principle at work. If we cut our finger, the blood will clot, and the wound will heal in time, of its own accord. In the same way, the naturopath would claim, the body will re-absorb an ulcer, or build new lung tissue, or heal an internal injury. It only needs to be allowed to get on with the job, unhampered by attempts to help, which are in reality no help at all, but simply acts which thwart its efforts. Drugs, as we have seen, just drive poisons deeper into the system, as well as adding to them. Surgery causes even greater injury than is there already, and adds to the healing that has to take place.

The naturopath uses a number of methods to help the body heal itself, and to help it to remain healthy when healed. They are: fasting, dieting, hydrotherapy, hygiene, psychotherapy, massage and sunshine. We shall look at each in turn.

FASTING

We all know that when a pet animal is ill, it will immediately stop eating. We know that when we are off colour, one of the first reactions is that we lose our appetite. These two facts alone should guide us to the theory that fasting is a natural first step in healing. It is more than that; it is one of the most important of the curative measures, because it gives the body an opportunity for self-cleansing. As long as we continue eating, we are simply adding to the store of waste products in our body all the time. As soon as we stop eating, elimination of those waste products speeds up. All the body's energies become free to work at the self-cleansing process.

The naturopath will certainly tell his patient to begin the treatment with a fast. This may last a couple of days or for some weeks. It should never be embarked on alone, as a form of self-treatment, but always after proper advice and under supervision. The longer fasts are normally only recommended for in-patients at Nature Cure institutions. Sometimes, during a fast, a patient will be asked to drink only water; sometimes he will be allowed fruit or vegetable juices. These drinks are taken at two hourly intervals, and they clean the digestive tracts and supply essential minerals to the body.

The first result of a fast is that the tongue becomes coated, the body temperature drops, and the patient may feel weak. This means that the cleansing process has begun. The furring of the tongue is cleansed by scraping it away with a wooden spatula. Fasting, it should be noted, is not starving. During the period of the fast, the body will live on stored surplus material. Toxins and waste matter that have accumulated in the tissues for years will start circulating, and hence they will be eliminated. When the tongue becomes clear again, it is time to end the fast. One point that must be guarded against is that the bowel action will become suspended during a fast. This is overcome by using a warm water enema daily to cleanse the bowels.

DIET

Naturopaths proceed from the viewpoint that we eat in order to live, not the other way round. There is no excuse for gluttony or for insisting on those foods we like in the way we like them. We must put health first. In their endeavour to make foods more pleasing to customers, manufacturers have refined and demineralised them. White bread and white rice are two good examples. Roughage has been taken out in the form of bran and husks; chemicals have been put in. The main drawback to such processing of food is that, apart from the additives that colour or preserve them, the mineral salts present in natural unprocessed foods have been lost, and these mineral salts are necessary for the body's cleansing and purifying system. The first step in planning diet, therefore, is to get back to fresh natural foods, such as fruit, vegetables, salads, and nuts, and to rely purely on foods that have been organically grown, so that they have not been affected by the sprays, fertilisers, and chemicals used on farms.

Conventional foods today, particularly white bread, white sugar, potatoes and meat, overload the system with acid waste. For proper functioning, the body and the blood must be alkaline. So the first step in the naturopathic diet is to restore lost alkalinity. Raw ripe fruit and vegetables will do this. Meat is not considered a good food at all. It is acid forming, liable to putrefy in the intestines, and suffers from the fact that the animal that produced it will undoubtedly have grazed on chemically treated grass, as well as having been injected against various diseases. Butter, cream, olive oil, dairy products in general and nuts are always to be preferred to meat. Brown sugar or honey or molasses are to be preferred to white sugar. Whole-meal bread still contains the roughage that is absent in the modern white loaf. Potatoes should be cooked in their skins. Condiments, sauces, spices, pastry, jam, puddings, tea, coffee, and alcohol should all be avoided. In addition to all this, the patient should not drink with meals, as this will dilute the digestive juices; he should take all his drinks between mealtimes.

Apart from general diet to preserve good health, the naturopath has special diets which he uses in treatments. After the initial fast, most patients will progress to the "All-Fruit Diet". This restores the alkalinity of the system, and builds up the patient's essential mineral salts. If, for any reason, a patient cannot take fruit, he will be given a raw vegetable diet instead. Sometimes the patient will be given the "Restricted Diet". This serves the same purpose as the All-Fruit Diet, but adds salads to the fruit. In both these diets, the fruit and the vegetables are eaten raw. The next step, following the fast and one or other of these diets, is to go onto the "Fruit and Milk Diet". The milk used in this must never be boiled but must be taken naturally. This diet begins to build the patient up, whilst the fruit is continuing the cleansing process. After a protracted fast under supervision, a patient may be put onto the "Full Milk Diet". Milk in its natural state is drunk in increasing quantities, the patient taking no other nourishment, but building up his intake under supervision.

All these diets are temporary and part of the general treatment. As soon as the patient recovers his health, he must go back onto a properly balanced diet, based on the principles detailed earlier.

HYDROTHERAPY

Various uses of hot and cold water are made by the naturopath. During fasting, as we have seen, the warm water enema is used to replace normal bowel functioning. This may be used at any time when the bowels are sluggish, and it is much preferred to drugs, which simply lash the bowels into fierce activity. This is the only internal use of water by the naturopath, and of course, enemas must not be used continuously. They are a temporary and emergency measure, until proper functioning is restored.

Sitz baths are used to re-vitalise the system. The principle of these is that the patient sits alternately in hot and cold water. Hot Epsom salt baths are sometimes prescribed as a cleansing agent, though they must be avoided in the case of patients with a weak heart. Warm baths generally are used to relax the patient, and may be combined with some of the treatments detailed in the chapter on Aroma therapy.

Another use of water is the wet pack. Cold packs are made by wringing out linen that has been soaked in cold water. They are then applied to the area of the body under treatment, which is afterwards covered with warm flannel. Cold packs will draw out inflammation and pain or reduce swelling.

Hot fomentations on the other hand soothe rheumatism or neuralgia. Other techniques of hydrotherapy are herbal baths, a salt rub applied when lying in a warm bath, sponging, under-water massage, and sprays.

Obviously, pure water is the most natural drink for man. It is always recommended in naturopathic practice, as an alternative to tea or coffee which are stimulants.

HYGIENE

By hygiene, the naturopath means not only what is commonly called cleanliness; that goes without saying; he also means getting plenty of fresh air, exercising, having adequate rest, and dressing sensibly. The patient should always sleep with his window open; he should get out into the fresh air as often as possible, preferably going into the country or to the seaside, where the pollution of city air is left behind; he should get used to breathing deeply.

Exercise does not necessarily mean physical jerks or sport; it simply means using your muscles. Walk instead of taking the car everywhere; do some gardening instead of watching TV every evening. Movement is life. Sedentary workers in particular must make sure that they have some activity that works their muscles gently and regularly, since mucles that are not used will tend to atrophy.

Rest is a part of hygiene. Avoid over-exhaustion. The human body needs about seven to eight hours sleep a night. Regular hours will establish a rhythm, and make getting to sleep easier. Tight nightclothes should be avoided, and nude sleeping is the best way of promoting deep rest. Early nights and early rising are conducive to health.

Dress is another consideration, and is often overlooked. The body needs to breathe, not only through the nose, but also through the pores of the skin. Loose clothing assists this. Tight collars and ties, though demanded by convention in certain occupations, should be discarded as soon as the wearer can, since they restrict the breathing. Boots and shoes have been called "coffins for the feet". They should certainly be well fitting and comfortable, and ladies should avoid high heels which throw the weight onto the toes, but everyone should try to go barefoot at some time in the day. One authority says that this earths electricity in the body, but whether this is true or not, the feet will benefit from the freedom. Although of course hereditary factors come into baldness, it is a fact that the wearing of hats also contributes.

Going without clothes altogether when possible is health-giving. The climate in Britain prevents nudism from becoming well-established, but to expose the whole body to the air for at least a part of each day will tone up the skin and promote relaxation and well-being.

PSYCHOTHERAPY

Naturopaths recognise that mental and physical factors intertwine. Mental and emotional states affect physical health. Worry is a potent factor in undermining any patient's resistance to disease. Psychotherapy will therefore play a part in any naturopathic treatment. The practitioner may use auto-suggestion, applied psychology, or just plain common-sense. If a patient is neurotic and could benefit from psycho-analysis or similar treatment, a naturopathic practitioner will refer him to a competent psychiatrist. Naturopaths insist, however, that psychotherapy on its own will not achieve results; there must be a review of the physical factors in the case as well.

MASSAGE

Massage helps to force toxic matter out of the areas of the body under treatment, so that it is carried around in the blood stream and eventually eliminated via the kidneys. Naturopaths use this form of treatment extensively, therefore, but always in conjunction with all the foregoing treatments.

SUNSHINE

The therapeutic value of sunshine to the body is inestimable. The sun promotes the growth of every living thing; it is a source of Vitamin D; it tones up the skin. Of course, it is important not to overdo sunbathing, and too much exposure can lead to skin cancer. A few minutes sunbathing each day are sufficient to begin with, gradually increasing the time as the skin bronzes over. Because of the limited amount of natural sunshine experienced in Britain, naturopaths make use of sun lamps in their treatment. With these it is most important not to over-expose the patient, and they should only be used by qualified practitioners, and goggles be provided for the patient. The widespread craze for sunbeds and instant tans provided by unqualified personnel today has little to do with nature cure, and can have serious ill effects.

Sunlight, either real or artificial, cannot effect a cure on its own, of course. It must always be used as an auxiliary to the other treatments to have the best results.

What conditions can naturopathy or hydrotherapy best help? The answer is every case that has not advanced to the stage where surgical intervention has become imperative to save life. The underlying cause of disease is always the same: wrong living. The cure is therefore always the same: right living. That is the simple philosophy of naturopathy. Even conditions like diabetes will sometimes respond to nature cure. It should be made clear, however, that a patient on carefully measured doses of insulin should on no account give them up without medical authority. What does sometimes happen is that his doctor who is monitoring his dosage will find that after naturopathic treatment it may be possible to reduce the dose and even in some cases to discontinue it.

Qualified practitioners of Naturopathy do not advertise. They use the degrees N.D. or D.O., or both, and M.B.N.O.A. A register of such practitioners can be obtained from The British Naturopathic and Osteopathic Association, (for the address see the Appendix page 151) for a fee, or it can be consulted at many Public Libraries.

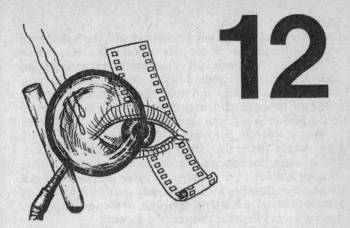

NEW DIAGNOSTIC METHODS

Orthodox doctors have various well-established methods of diagnosis. These include case history, taking of temperature, feeling of pulse, sounding with stethoscope, observing physical appearance, taking X-rays, analysing urine samples etc. Practitioners of alternative therapies have a few more methods to add to these. Reference has already been made to the twelve pulses which an acupuncturist claims to be able to feel, and the four qualities that a hakim will detect. The other diagnostic techniques which are used mainly or exclusively by practitioners of alternative medicine are: dowsing, hair analysis, iridiology, and Kirlian photography. They are particularly relevant to patients who are seeking healing without harm, since they harm neither patient nor animal. Some orthodox methods do. Exploratory surgery, for example, whilst having a beneficial intent, does harm the patient at the time. Some forms of pregnancy testing harm laboratory animals to which samples are given.

DOWSING

Probably most readers will be familiar with the forked twig with which some people are able to find water. It is held in both hands and will tilt downwards to indicate an underground supply. Some dowsers use a pendulum instead, and in the chapters on Faith Healing and Radionics, we look at the use of the pendulum to detect illness in greater detail. In the Middle Ages, such methods would have been looked upon as witchcraft, but healers today feel that they are only using natural forces that have not yet been fully understood. Just as some dowsers seeking water can find it by holding their pendulum over a map, so some practitioners can diagnose by dowsing without actually seeing the patient. A sample of blood, a few strands of hair, or even a photograph are sufficient to enable this method to work.

HAIR ANALYSIS

This method of diagnosis is based upon the fact that the nutritional state of our hair reflects the nutritional state of our body, and hence any mineral deficiency in the latter will show up in a hair sample. The patient is asked to supply about one gram of hair, which is roughly two tablespoonfuls, cut as near the scalp as possible. This sample is analysed using atomic emission spectroscopy, to find out the levels of twenty-two minerals in it. Since hair grows at about the rate of half an inch a month, hair one and a half inches long will give average body mineral levels for the past three months. This will show if there is any deficiency or imbalance. Hair analysts will then discuss with their patient the function of each mineral in the body, and how he may remedy any deficiency before it leads to illness. This can sometimes be done by supplements to an existing diet, or by a change of diet. The technique is thus particularly useful for forecasting what might go wrong, and for taking preventive measures in time.

IRIDIOLOGY

Iridiology is more widely used than either of the above methods. We all know that when we visit the optician, his examination of our eyes can reveal other conditions in the body, and he will sometimes advise a visit to the doctor. Iridiology is an extension of this observation. The use of eye examination for specific diagnoses dates back to the early 1800's. A Hungarian boy, Ignatz von Peczely, caught an owl and accidentally broke its leg. He noticed that this led to a black stripe arising in the owl's eye. As he nursed the owl back to health, he observed that this black stripe dwindled to a speck and disappeared when the owl was better. Growing up to be a physician, von Peczely remembered the owl, and began to study the irises of accident victims, and people who underwent surgery. He saw that the irises mirrored changes in the various organs, and thus began the science of iridiology.

It is in the eye that the nervous system comes to the surface, and the iris reflects all parts of the body, and even the mind and the spirit. The lines, flecks, and pigments guide the iridiologist not only to what is wrong at the moment of examination but also to what may have been wrong in the past or may go wrong in the future. It should be said, however, that it does not show up specific illnesses; rather it indicates the things a patient may be prone to. Congestion of the digestive system, circulation problems, stomach acidity, tendency to a weak heart, these are the kind of things that show up, and they may develop into problems or they may not. At least the pin-pointing of the danger spots and signals can alert the patient, so that he can take preventative measures.

Iridiology is used by some osteopaths, acupuncturists, herbalists, and homoeopaths, and even if they do not specialise in iridiology themselves, they may refer patients for this type of examination.

In earlier times, this examination would have been lengthy. The patient would have had to sit, eyes wide open, whilst the iridiologist carried out the examination with a magnifying glass and a torch. Today, the iridiologist photographs each eye, using a special camera, and then makes slides which he can project onto a screen, and compare with charts of the iris. This diagnostic method commends itself to patients, for three reasons: it is quick; it is painless; and it is completely safe. From the practitioner's point of view, it has the advantage that he can learn all about his patient in one go.

The left iris corresponds with the left side of the body, the right with the right side. At the top of the iris information relating to the brain and the head is to be found; in the centre the stomach and the organs of digestion; moving outwards, indications are given as to the intestines and the colon; still further, the kidneys, the liver, the back, and the skin. Bluish rings round the outer rim of the iris can show stress problems; pupil size is related to nervous response; textural appearance indicates recuperative ability. The iridiologist has detailed charts with which to compare the photographic slides he has made.

Iridiologists do not generally treat patients themselves, unless they are also practitioners of one of the alternative therapies. They see their work as indicating to the practitioner the risk areas. A course in the skill is run by The School of Iridiology and Wholistic Healing (for the address see the Appendix page 151) but as yet there are no professional qualifications.

KIRLIAN PHOTOGRAPHY

Kirlian photography still needs a lot of investigation and research before it becomes a reliable diagnostic tool, but it has very interesting possibilities for the future. It is a technique of high frequency photography, named after its inventors, Semyon and Valentian Kirlian. Briefly, the apparatus used consists of an insulated aluminium plate on top of a box in which is a high frequency electrical coil. On top of the aluminium plate is placed a glass plate, a sheet of photographic film unexposed, then a sheet of protective plastic. The object to be photographed is pressed onto the plastic sheet, a current is passed through the apparatus for a few seconds, and energy emitted by the object interacts with the electric current to produce an image on the photographic film.

The images thus produced are marks that apparently emanate from the object, and they correspond with the aura which psychics claim they can see around people. Some researchers will not concede that there is anything supernatural or spiritual about this aura. They account for it purely in terms of electro-magnetic and thermal fields surrounding the object. Psychics can see this without any apparatus; Kirlian photography reveals it to all.

Be the explanation what it may, the aura that the Kirlian method detects appears as sparks emanating from the object, and the pattern of the emanations and their colours can be used as a diagnostic tool for detecting physical and mental disorders, even before any other symptoms appear. Using a leaf, for example, it has been found that a plant disease can be detected before any other method of examination will reveal it. When a leaf withers, the colours in the aura fade, and Semyon Kirlian found that when he was ill, the pictures of his hands became blurred and cloudy.

Most of the research up to the present has been carried out in the Soviet Union, but the West is now engaged in the study as well. Photographs of the hands of a patient immediately before a session with a healer show a less clear aura than after, which suggests a higher level of energy in the "healed" patient. Hands that have been photographed before and after a yoga session also show a clearer aura afterwards, suggesting that the yoga has benefited the patient. This effect has not been noticed after a session at any other sport, however.

A fascinating aspect of this subject is that when Russian researchers cut off a portion of a leaf, they were still getting a picture of the aura of the whole. Thelma Moss, who is engaged in research in the U.S.A., records in her book "The Body Electric" that despite many attempts, her team were only once able to do this. But if with improved apparatus or technique, the Russian success could be duplicated with regularity, the implications even in the philosophical and religious fields are tremendous. It would suggest that all living things, whether vegetable or animal, have a psychic body, permeating and duplicating their physical body, as spiritualists have always claimed. More importantly, it would suggest that this psychic body is not mutilated by mutilation of the physical body, but retains its wholeness. It would make the religious doctrine of the resurrection of the body understandable, since the psychic body is incorruptible.

Once a leaf or an animal has died, the aura detected by Kirlian photography fades. This again accords with the idea of the spiritual or psychic body leaving the physical body at death. Non-living objects, such as coins, keys etc. do not have an aura.

Those people gifted with the ability to see a person's aura without any apparatus have usually claimed that they were able to tell from the aura whether or not the person was in good health. Kirlian photography could provide this information by mechanical means, doing away with the intermediary of the person who can see auras, and overcoming the subjectivity of observations based on what this person saw.

When a woman was photographed at various times during the menstrual cycle, her fingers showed a more pronounced aura at the time of ovulation. Kirlian enthusiasts have claimed that cancer can be detected at an early stage by studying the aura. One application that has been suggested for the future is to test, by the variation in the aura, whether a therapist is giving the right treatment to a patient. This would be a quick guide, and enable treatment to be changed at once, if necessary, rather than after a month or so, as is done with homoeopathic treatments.

Obviously, much more needs to be done before this technique becomes a standard diagnostic method. It could well be a tool of the future, however.

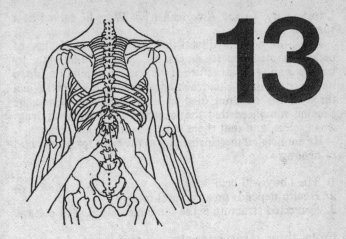

OSTEOPATHY

Like chiropractic, osteopathy has its roots in the manipulative treatments of the Chinese and the Egyptians, and the writings of Hippocrates and the ancient Greeks. Such skills were also known to Red Indians, to the Russians, to Dr. Hermann Boerhaave, a Dutchman, in the seventeenth century, and to English bone-setters even earlier. But osteopathy, as it is practised today, was started at the end of the nineteenth century by Dr. Andrew Taylor Still.

Dr. Still was born in Virginia, North America, in 1828. He was the son of a Methodist missionary, who was also qualified as a doctor. Missionaries, particularly in frontier settlements, often combined both functions in those days. Andrew Taylor Still first studied medicine under his father. Again, this method of training was quite common before medical colleges came into being. He did later complete his studies at The College of Physicians and Surgeons, in

Kansas City. In the American Civil War, he served as a surgeon.

Dr. Still became dissatisfied with the approaches of orthodox medicine to illness. He believed that only by understanding the structure of the body in its relationship to its use could there be a true understanding of illness. When three of his children died in a meningitis epidemic, he became convinced that the standard treatment with drugs was useless, and that there must be some other way.

He enunciated three principles as the basis for his method of healing:

1. The body will heal itself.
2. Health depends on structural integrity.
3. Perverted structure is the fundamental cause of disease.

From these three principles, he developed the art of osteopathy, which is a manipulative therapy.

One of Dr. Still's early cases was a child suffering with dysentery. He relates that when he placed his hand on the child's body, he found that it was warm in the lumbar region, but cold on the stomach; again, the back of the head and neck were warm, but the face was cold. His first thought was to try to move heat from the warm to the cold places, and he began pressing and rubbing. In so doing, he found that in places the body felt loose and flabby, whereas at other spots it felt firm and congested.

He went on to work on the child's spine, and felt abnormalities there, which he proceeded to adjust. These abnormalities he called "osteopathic lesions", a term that provoked a great deal of abuse from orthodox circles, in the early days. Doubt was even expressed as to the existence of these lesions. Today, osteopaths call them "areas of somatic disfunction".

The simple techniques that Dr. Still used on the child cured him in one session, though dysentery was often a killer disease in those days. From this simple beginning, Dr. Still came to understand how, by simply feeling a patient's body, he could detect abnormalities, and by manipulation he could restore normal functions. He began to have success with asthma and pneumonia, and as he did so, his fame spread.

In 1892, he founded the first College of Osteopathy in Kirksville. Today, there are twelve schools in the United States, and graduates in America have exactly the same status as ordinary doctors. They can practise any form of medicine as well as osteopathic techniques; they can sign death certificates. The position in Britain and in other countries is less happy, however.

The philosophy of osteopathy is a holistic one, like so many other of the alternative therapies. The whole man in his environment must be considered. Disease is defined as the disparity between the demands made upon an individual by his work, his play, social conditions and stress, and his capacity to respond to those demands. He is not to be thought of as "ill" simply because he has some condition known as a "disease"; he has this disease because he is ill, that is, his body is not coping with the demands made upon it.

Two schools of thought have long persisted in medicine. One is that outside forces enter the body to cause disease; the other that forces inside the body are responsible. There is evidence in favour of both theories. We know that we can catch contagious diseases from exposure to germs; we know too that internal weaknesses can make us ill. However, osteopaths tend to believe that unless the body is weakened by internal stresses, its resistance would be sufficient to combat oustide attacks. Left alone, the body will naturally tend to heal itself; it must be helped, not hindered with drugs. And this is one of the basic teachings of osteopathy.

Osteopaths believe that any disturbance in the mechanical or bone structure of the body will put organs and their functions under strain. In this they are at one with chiropractors, and like them they pay a great deal of attention to the spine, and the nerve system that it houses.

The spinal cord is the most important channel for nerves in the body. Every movement and every function of the body is controlled through this channel. If a nerve is trapped at its exit, the organ it serves will suffer, not only because messages from the brain to the organ are not getting through properly, but also because messages back from the organ to the brain are being affected as well. There is a two way traffic, and the body's reaction to any blockage of the channel is to make the messages even more strident. This makes the point where the nerve is trapped even more sensitive.

Osteopaths lay great stress on correct posture, whether standing up, seated, or even lying down. Faulty posture increases the strain on the spine. Osteopaths recognise that the nervous system not only carries messages from the brain to different parts of the body; it also governs the transportation of protein, fat and other nutrients. Any hindrance to the nervous system can, therefore, lead to the degenerative diseases. They know that restriction of a joint's movement will not only affect surrounding tissues, but will impede circulation and the work of more distant organs. They know that breathing is important to a patient's well-being, since not only does it provide oxygen for the body but it assists elimination. It is important, therefore, that no bone misalignment interferes with correct breathing.

The osteopath is popularly thought of as a man who puts bones back into place, a simple bone-setter, but his work is much more comprehensive than this. He certainly does restore bones to place, and normalizes the range of movement in joints, but he also uses many other techniques in his treatment.

He will massage tissue, sometimes with firm, sometimes with gentle pressure. He will improve range of movement in a faulty joint in three ways. Sometimes, he will make a sharp adjustment; sometimes, he will take the joint gently to the limit of its movement, and gradually increase it; sometimes he will hold it still and encourage the patient to try to move it against the resistance he is offering. He will be able to use points that trigger off a patient's reflex actions. He will sometimes use the technique of taking a joint into its easiest position and then subjecting it to a mild degree of strain in order to get a reflex release of congested tissue.

Apart from the practical techniques, the osteopath will advise his patient on any changes in life-style that may be necessary to enable his body to cope without falling into the same condition again. Osteopathy is a preventive medicine. In this counselling, the practitioner is mainly concerned to remove stress from the patient's life, be it physical or mental.

Training in Britain is rather different from that in the United States, where a seven year general medical course is normal. In Britain, there are three Colleges:

The British School of Osteopathy, The British College of Osteopathy and Naturopathy, and The European School of Osteopathy, (for their addresses see the Appendix page 151).

These colleges offer a full-time four-year course that leads to the degrees of M.R.O., M.B.N.O.A., or M.S.O. respectively. Surgery and pharmacology do not form part of the courses in British colleges, but the London School of Osteopathy does offer a one-year course to qualified medical practitioners, and after taking this, they would of course be on a par with their American counterparts.

Unfortunately, there is no statutory registration of osteopaths in Britain, so that it is open to anyone, with little or no qualification, to call himself an osteopath. This situation adversely affects the qualified man, since he is not allowed to advertise, whereas the unqualified practitioner can and frequently does.

Doctors are beginning to realise that properly trained osteopaths have their part to play in patient care, and some osteopaths work in hospitals or have patients referred to them by the medical profession. On the whole, though, the medical profession tends to regard osteopathy as an auxiliary to be called in after the doctor has made the diagnosis; osteopaths themselves would assert that they are doctors in their own right and capable of doing their own diagnosis.

The methods they use in diagnosis are: to observe changes in the symmetry of the body, which to them will indicate displacement of a bone or bone segment; to note restrictions in the mobility of a joint or limb; and to look out for changes in the texture of tissue. Their first test is usually palpation, that is feeling the body, or various parts of it, with their hands. From his touch, the trained osteopath can find problem areas, just as Dr. Still did with his dysentery patient. They will then try to get the patient to move, in order to assess range and ease of movement in various limbs and joints.

Osteopaths are especially trained to look out for what they call "soft tissue changes", that is tension in the skin, hard areas, change in temperature at a specific point, tenderness, or excessive fluid. A highly developed sense of touch is needed for this kind of examination, but once the osteopath has developed this ability, palpation will tell him things that the patient may not even remember himself about past illnesses.

If it is felt necessary, X-rays may be used as part of the diagnosing. The heart, the chest, the blood pressure and urine samples may also be examined in some cases. All these things, together with the patient's past medical history and his present life-style will combine to tell the practitioner what is wrong.

Treatment usually begins with soft tissue manipulation. This is a kind of stretching, massaging movement, that is both pleasant and relaxing. If there has to be joint manipulation to follow, this is usually carried out with a short sharp thrust, which may produce a click as something goes back into place. This click often reassures patients that things are now put right, but it is not always heard, and the patient should not be dismayed if he does not notice it. The thrust itself is nothing to be feared; it is normally quite painless and quick.

An osteopath will always discuss with his patient exactly what has to be done, and this of itself breeds confidence. The secrecy that seems part of orthodox medical practice is completely absent when you consult an osteopath or indeed any of the alternative practitioners.

What conditions are likely to benefit from osteopathic treatment? Most people go in the first place for back troubles, including the so-called "slipped disc". Back troubles are often baffling to the orthodox medical practitioner, and surgery or traction often makes matters worse. Other conditions that respond very well to osteopathy are: rheumatism, arthritis, migraine, tension, headaches, bronchitis, and menstrual problems. Allergic conditions, constipation, varicose veins, cystitis, infertility, and impotence have sometimes been helped. False angina, in which the patient feels the classic symptoms without actually having the disease, can often be made to disappear. Hiatus hernia symptoms can be minimized. It has been known for osteopathy to take away the need for an operation.

Recently, there has been a new development in the treatment known as cranial manipulation. The bones of the skull have been found to move slightly with breathing, and it is claimed that this movement carries out a circulatory function in the intricate channels surrounding the brain. An extremely gentle treatment can be applied to this area. The practitioner will simply hold the bones with his hands, whilst the patient's own breathing improves their positioning and function.

Conditions that have resulted from a blow to the head, such as tinnitus, Menière's disease, and visual disturbances, can sometimes be helped by this treatment. It is also used with premature babies. If a premature baby is refusing food, cries too much, does not sleep, or fails to show normal development, treatment by cranial manipulation can sometimes prevent more serious conditions from developing later on.

Apart from treatment for a particular condition, patients will see an osteopath for general health care. They will receive a general check-up, just as careful as an orthodox doctor would give them, and any slight problems revealed can then be put right before they develop. Often a patient's main need is for someone to listen to him, and he wants to talk to someone who is qualified to reassure him. A good osteopath has both the time and the medical expertise to do both.

In a profession where the poorly trained and the unqualified out-number the genuine practitioners, it is wise to be careful in your choice of consultant. You cannot do better than to get the directory of qualified osteopaths available from The British School of Osteopathy (for the address, see the Appendix page 151).

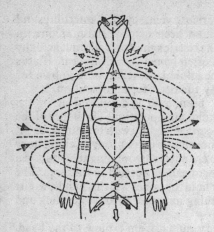

RADIONICS

Radionics like faith healing has affinities with dowsing (see page 106), in that it uses forces not fully understood. Some practitioners believe that what they are doing will be explained in purely scientific terms when man has greater knowledge; these see themselves as using purely natural laws. Others give their work a spiritual or psychic dimension, linking it with religious teachings of either East or West. Perhaps ultimately it is unhelpful to try to divide knowledge into compartments labelled natural and supernatural; rather should we see truth as a whole, though accepting that it can only partly be comprehended at present.

In the nineteenth century, it was discovered that dowsers could distinguish between pure and impure water by their rod, and could even identify different kinds of impurity. From this it was a short step to using dowsing instruments, and in particular the pendulum, to distinguish beween healthy and unhealthy parts of the body. The pendulum would have a different reaction when held over a healthy organ from what it had when held over an unhealthy one. Some practitioners took the technique a stage further. They would use it to choose the right remedies. By holding different homoeopathic remedies, one at a time, in one hand, and the pendulum in the other, they could tell from the pendulum's reaction which remedy to choose.

Diagnosis with a pendulum was developed in France by Abbé Mermet, at the end of the nineteenth century. He called the technique "radiesthesia". As he was a highly respected member of the Church, and had studied the subject very carefully and scientifically, his ideas gained acceptance in his own country and in Italy. Amongst those who consulted him was the Pope of his day. Britain and the United States were not so sympathetic in their reactions.

Radiesthesia owed its development in America to Dr. Albert Abrams. He had studied physics as well as medicine, and after completing his studies in Europe he became a neurologist of international renown. A purely chance experience with a patient started his research into radionics. Whilst he was giving a check-up to a patient who was suffering from an ulcer on the lip, Dr. Adams found that one small area of the patient's stomach sounded dull when tapped instead of hollow. This only happened, however, when the patient was facing west. Abrams deduced that this phenomenon had something to do with the earth's magnetic field.

He began examining patients suffering from various diseases, and came to the conclusion that atoms in diseased tissue emanated some kind of radiation. He was able to relate different sounding points to different diseases. He argued that if healthy and diseased tissue gave off different radiations, it should be possible to build equipment that would detect those radiations, diagnose the disease and cure it. From this research, he came to the conclusion that the basis of disease was electronic and hence that the cure would be electronic.

The apparatus he designed became popularly known as "the black box". It produced measured vibrations, which he claimed destroyed the infection in the patient. His work was scoffed at by some, but when it was tested by the British Medical Association in 1924, his claims for its success at diagnosis were upheld. However, even after this, Abrams did not receive recognition, since his opponents held that the machine that had been used in the tests was not in fact Dr. Abrams' but a later model. He died a disappointed man.

Following his death, Ruth Drown carried on his research. She was a chiropractor who had worked with Abrams. She discarded the use of electric currents in her machines, and used only the body's own energy for diagnosis and treatment. Abrams had already found that it was not necessary for a patient to be present in order to arrive at an accurate diagnosis. He could find out what was wrong from a blood spot alone. The blood spot was a microcosm, containing within it all the attributes of the macrocosm. Absent diagnosis and healing had become a possibility, since, by use of the blood spot, the machine could be tuned in to the distant patient. By focusing the healing vibrations on the blood spot, they could be sent forth to the distant patient. These were the striking claims of radionics.

Ruth Drown worked out a list of treatments for various illnesses, for use on her machine, and in the 1930's and 1940's, she had a large practice in America. In 1951, however, she was arrested on a charge of fraud and medical quackery, and it was ordered that her instruments be destroyed. Despite the evidence of people who said they had been cured, the practice of radionics was made illegal in most of the United States.

Investigation continued in Britain and in the Soviet Union and is still going on today. George de la Warr became interested in Britain, after he had been asked to build a copy of the Drown instrument. From the 1940's onwards, he and his wife began to design and manufacture new equipment. Their diagnostic instrument had nine knobs. The blood spot was placed in small cups. The operator would rotate the dials as he stroked a thin rubber membrane at the base of the instrument. When the membrane had a sticky feel, he would know that the correct reading had been set up. He had then only to look up the reading in a table of rates and the disease would be found. A separate but similar instrument was designed for treatment using the blood spot as a focus.

The basic concept of radionics is that man, in company with all other life forms, is submerged in the electro-magnetic energy field of the earth. Each life form has its own electro-magnetic field. Today, the modern scientific concept is that all is energy, even what we popularly think of as solid matter, since this consists of protons and electrons around a nucleus. Radionics sees all man's organs, diseases and remedies as having their own particular vibration or frequency, and these frequencies are expressed numerically as "rates", which can be set up on the dials of the machines. The link between patient and practitioner is provided by the earth's electro-magnetic field.

The practitioner uses extra-sensory perception rather as a dowser uses his rod. He attunes his mind to the distant patient when he puts the blood spot into his machine. He poses questions, but he is more concerned with the causes of his patient's condition rather that their physical manifestation. His aim is to help his patient to realise his full potential in life, and thereby find health and happiness. Like all the other therapies in this book, the aim is therefore holistic. Radionics sometimes becomes linked with spiritual beliefs, and practitioners will then have similar ideas to faith healers. They will see the patient and themselves as having etheric bodies linked in the vast sea of etheric energy.

Two other aspects of radionics were developed by Ruth Drown. They are radionic photography, and radionic potentising of remedies.

In radionic photography, no light reaches the photographic plate; it is activated by the life energy of the patient. We are familiar with the way in which X-rays can produce an image on a plate; in radionics we are being asked to go a step further and believe that emanations from the human body or from a blood spot can do the same thing. By this means, photographs of distant patients have been obtained from blood spots. In the 1950's the de la Warr Laboratories pressed ahead with investigation of radionic photography, using newly developed cameras, and with these, photographs were obtained which show the organs of the body very clearly.

One of the most interesting is of a patient with tuberculosis of the lung. Although this patient had only one lung when the photograph was taken, the other having been removed, both lungs show up in the picture. The tuberculosis appears as a white mass over the one lung, the other is a shadowy outline, but still there. When we compare this with the photograph obtained by Kirlian photography of a complete leaf when part had been cut away, the evidence for the existence of this etheric body they speak of, is mounting, as is the idea that it is unmutilated by mutilation of the physical body.

George de la Warr says: "In my experience of our radionic camera, the presence of a magnetic field indicates the presence of etheric energy. The magnetic fields of nature are completely suffused with the energy patterns of the etheric counterpart." He was in no doubt that the photographs he took were of the etheric body.

We have already seen in the chapters on The Bach Flower Remedies and on Homoeopathy how the healing powers of plants are potentised. Dr. Ruth Drown was the first radionic practitioner to prepare homoeopathic remedies by radionic means. Since her day, the de la Warr laboratories have produced a sophisticated electrically energised machine for doing this. The tincture of the remedy required is placed in one well of the machine; plain tablets, water, or alcohol, whichever is required, are placed in the other well. The rate representing the tincture is set up on the dials, and the machine switched on. In about twenty minutes, the unmedicated tablets, water or alcohol will have become impregnated with the potentisation of the tincture in the other well. A further development of this process, invented by Malcolm Ray is the Ray Potency Simulator. This uses simulator cards instead of the tincture in order to potentise sal lac tablets.

Like chiropractors and osteopaths, radionic practitioners are well aware of the importance of the spine to health, and an engineer, Darrel Butcher, who became interested in radionics in the 1950's, designed an instrument known as the Peggoty Board. This treats spinal disorders at a distance, working from a blood sample. Pegs are placed in a board to set up the healing rate required, which is obtained from charts.

Radionic practitioners claim to be able to help any condition in a patient, or, if they are not or feel that the patient would do better with another form of treatment, they are ready to refer such patients to chiropractors or homoeopaths.

A certain degree of faith is needed to seek radionic treatment. Scepticism can limit its effectiveness, and to the man-in-the-street, the idea that illness can be diagnosed at a distance from a blood spot and healing sent forth with only the focused attention of the practitioner to provide the link may sound too far-fetched for credibility. So would television or flight to the moon have sounded to our grandparents. It is worth approaching the subject with an open mind.

To find a qualified radionic practitioner, consult The Radionic Association (for the address see the Appendix page 151). They run a two year course, which leads to the qualification M.RAD.A., member of the Radionics Association, and a further course leading to the Fellowship, F.RAD.A. They also keep a register of qualified members.

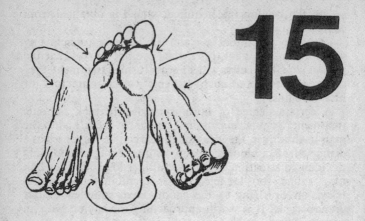

15

REFLEXOLOGY

Reflexology is a system of diagnosis and healing by massaging the feet. It depends on links between certain areas of the feet and organs of the body. Foot massage is believed to have been practised by the ancient Chinese and Egyptian civilisations, but reflexology in the form that we know it today dates from the nineteen-twenties, when Dr. Fitzgerald, an American, and some of his colleagues started relating various zones of the body to sensitive areas on the feet.

Dr. Fitzgerald's studies were triggered off when he noticed that patients would sometimes clutch parts of their feet when they experienced symptoms, or even when they were anxious. His work on this was taken up and developed more fully by another American, Miss Eunice D. Ingham, and it was she who actually mapped out the sensitive areas on the toes, the sole and the ankles of each foot. An English nurse visiting America became so interested in these ideas that she studied under Miss Ingham before returning to Britain to introduce the techniques here. She was Miss Doreen E. Bayley, and she set up The Bayley School of Reflexology. When she died in 1979, Nicola Hall became the head of the School.

Reflexology is sometimes known as "compression massage". The patient is made comfortable, either in a reclining chair or on a treatment couch. Pillows are placed under the head and the knees. He is encouraged to relax. If the patient is unable to visit the practitioner and is being treated at home, conditions as near as possible to these will be created. An easy chair for the patient, with another chair or stool on which to rest his feet, will usually suffice. The practitioner himself will sit on a low stool at the feet of the patient, facing them, whilst he carries out the treatment.

Both the thumb and the fingers are used for the massage. It begins at the toes, and is rather like a creeping forwards of the finger-tips moving down the sole of the foot. It could be compared to a many legged insect walking down. Some patients think they can feel the reflexologist's nails digging into their feet, but, of course, he is careful to keep them trimmed short and this is most unlikely to be the case.

Areas of the feet are related to parts of the body. The toes correspond to the top of the head. The hollows at the base of the toes are the ears and eyes. The sides of the foot by the little toes represent the shoulders. Lower down on the foot are the thyroid, the lungs, the heart. Still lower, are the solar plexus, the stomach and the spleen. About half way down the foot, is the waist line, the kidneys and the transverse colon, and below it, the descending colon and the small intestine. The heel corresponds to the sciatic area. The sides of the heel represent the hip and the lower back. The back of the ankle gives the rectum and the prostate gland. Points on the side of the foot represent the ovaries or the testicles. On top of the foot is found the breast area, with the bronchial and lung areas.

Detailed charts make all this clear to practitioner and patient. They were drawn up by Doreen Bayley, and though there are now several different schools of thought in the work, these charts have not changed since her day. They are really just commonsense. If we look at the soles of someone's feet, side by side, and think of them as corresponding to the body, the head is naturally at the top. The right foot corresponds to the right side of the body, the left foot to the left side, so some organs will occur in one foot, others in the other, and a few will spread across both feet, as they do in the torso.

When treating a patient, the reflexologist will normally only spend ten minutes on each foot at the first session, lengthening it gradually to about half an hour. If he finds any special areas of tenderness or pain, he would be careful not to give them too much massage at first, but might return to them at the end of a session. He would, however, take careful note where such areas were, as clearly they speak of conditions of the body. At the end of each session, the reflexologist has a special way of relaxing the patient. He will press on the solar plexus reflex in the foot, and gently move the foot in time with the patient's breathing.

How does reflexology work? No-one really knows. Reflexologists tend to reject the idea that their therapy is linked with acupressure and that what they are really doing is restoring the balance of yin and yang. Their usual theory is that they are breaking up and dispersing crystals in the reflexes, which are causing congestion and interfering with the blood's circulation. Some believe that their massage triggers off an electrical impulse, and that energy flows to revitalise the patient. Some link their work with the belief in an etheric body, and claim that they are bringing about a state of harmony between the physical and the etheric body. How reflexology works is as puzzling as some of the other therapies; the fact that it does work in some cases is indisputable. We are, once again, on the frontier of human knowledge.

Reflexes are also found on a patient's hands. The brain is at the ends of the thumbs; the eyes at the base of the first and second fingers; the ears at the base of the third and fourth fingers; the shoulder reflex is a point just below the little finger; the lungs and heart lie below the two middle fingers; the solar plexus, the spleen and the colon are all lower down the hand; the ovaries or testicles are on the little finger edge of the hands at the bottom; the sciatic area is just above the wrist. On the back of the hands, the upper lymphatic area is at the base of the fingers; the heart reflex in the middle of the hand; the arms and groin at the sides and base of the hand. All these points are again mapped out on charts and roughly correspond to what would be expected, if you look at the palms or the backs of your hands and think of them as the torso.

Hand reflexes can be massaged in exactly the same way as foot reflexes. Indeed, if the foot has been amputated, it is the hand that the reflexologist will have to work on. Treatment on the hand is not quite as effective as that given on the foot, however.

Lines known as "zones" link areas in the body. They run from the top of the head down each side of the body to link up with the end of each toe and each finger. There are thus ten on each side of the body. Along these lines a flow of energy joins organs in the path. They are not nerve pathways or veins or arteries, and some would say that, like the meridians of Ch'i, they are fictional. They do not, however, correspond to the meridians of Ch'i, in positioning.

Besides these lines, there are cross reflexes. These can be found between elbow and knee; between shoulder and hip, between hand and foot, and in other places. Pain is often felt at a distance from its point of origin. It is then known as referred pain. Using his knowledge of the cross reflexes, a reflexologist can bring relief. A damaged wrist may lead to pain in the ankle. Massage of the ankle would then bring relief to the wrist.

Reflexology, as has been indicated, can be used for diagnosis as well as treatment. By testing the degree of tenderness in the reflex areas, the reflexologist can quickly pin-point organs that are in trouble. The method is painless, quick and accurate, in the hands of a properly trained man, with the necessary knowledge of anatomy and physiology.

Among the disorders that reflexology treats are: migraine, polio, glaucoma, cataract, deafness, head injuries and cerebral haemorrhage, which are treated through massage of the toes; spinal troubles such as old injuries and what are commonly called "slipped discs", which are treated through massage of the spinal reflexes; thyroid troubles, heart, lung complaints, asthma, kidney trouble, liver, gall bladder, prostate troubles, neuritis, arthritis, all of which respond to massage of the appropriate reflexes. There is no condition that reflexology does not claim to help, though it does not pretend to be a cure-all on its own, and is frequently combined with other treatments, so how much of the cure is due to reflexology and how much to the other therapy is a matter for conjecture. Only in one case should reflexology not be tried. This is thrombosis, where massage might stimulate movement of the blood clot rather than dispersal, with fatal results perhaps.

Reflexology suffers, perhaps unjustly, in the public estimation, because too many who call themselves "reflexologists" have simply learnt from a text book or correspondence course or at a short weekend course. It is true that the actual techniques can be learnt very quickly, because they are simple. Perhaps a short introductory course would enable a student to treat himself, or to practise on his family without much harm. But the public demand something more than this from a man whom they consult, and to whom they pay a fee. This extra training is also being demanded by the International Institute of Reflexology, so that a higher status will be given to the treatment. The Institute demands that a student should pass both a written and an oral examination, and should do practical work under supervision before he qualifies. It also runs advanced courses to keep the practitioner up-to-date with latest developments, and to teach him about other therapies which he could recommend to the patient if necessary.

Courses in reflexology and further information can be obtained from The Bayley School of Reflexology, or from The International Institute of Reflexology. Reflexology charts can be bought from The Crusade Against All Cruelty to Animals Ltd., (for their addresses see the Appendix page 152).

It will be realised from this that no harmful use of animals is made either in the training of practitioners or in research, and hence reflexology will appeal as a form of treatment to those who oppose vivisection or the use of animals in drug testing. Reflexology is truly healing without harm.

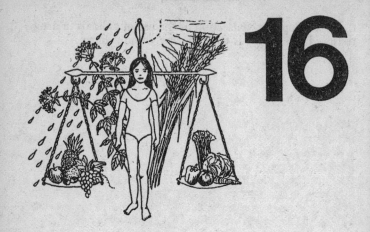

SELF HELP

Self Help is the oldest of all the alternative therapies. Before the advent of free medicine in Britain, it was widely practised by people too poor to pay the doctor. In many parts of the world today it is the only medicine readily available. Even if you qualify for National Health Service treatment, or are in a private scheme, it is still in your interest to do as much as you can for yourself. As we have seen, the drug-based therapy of orthodox medicine is not always the best treatment.

There are five main areas in which you can do something to keep your body in good health: a balanced diet, adequate exercise, avoidance of stress, watching your weight, and practising relaxation. We have touched on some of these already, particularly in connection with naturopathy, but it is worth looking again at them in the light of what you can do yourself. If having taken all precautions, you do succumb to some minor ailment, consider self-treatment with herbal remedies rather than rushing to the doctor.

BALANCED DIET

The nutritional requirements of the human body can be divided into seven groups: proteins, carbohydrates, fats, minerals, vitamins, roughage, and other elements. We get these things from the food we eat, and it is therefore important to eat the right food in the right quantity. Unfortunately, as we have already seen, many of our foods have been chemically treated or processed to such an extent that they have lost their nutritional value. Crop sprays and fertilisers have left their traces in our food, and these can affect our health adversely. It is wise to eat as much organically grown and unprocessed, unpreserved food as we can.

Our bodies consist of countless cells, all of which are made of protein and require protein for their repair and replacement. These cells are renewed once every seven years. Protein is found in meat, fish, eggs, milk, peas, beans, cheese, and bread. An active young man will need 90g per day, a moderately active one 75g, and one pursuing a sedentary occupation 70g. The female requirement is 12g less than the male, except during pregnancy, when it is the same. The figures decrease to about 55g per day as old age approaches.

Carbohydrates with fats give us energy, and the unit of energy in dietary considerations is the calorie. The commonest sources of carbohydrates are sugar, fruit, honey, flour, bread, cereals, potatoes, rice, semolina, lentils and beans. An active man needs 3600 calories per day, a moderately active one 3000, and a sedentary worker 2700. A very active woman needs 2500, but 2200 is the normal for the female, except in pregnancy, when between 200 and 500 extra calories are needed. The figures all drop to about 2000 in old age. Fats and carbohydrates must be counted together as energy sources, though fats give us more than just energy. They assist growth; they insulate the body against cold; and they make food more palatable.

Minerals help the growth and repair of the body. We need

calcium to build and maintain our bones and teeth. 800mg per day is the requirement for either a man or a woman, but during pregnancy, the woman may need as much as 1200mg. These figures decrease to 500mg in old age. Calcium is found in milk, cheese, cereals and bread. We need iron for the red corpuscles of the blood. 12mg per day is needed for a man or woman, except during pregnancy, when the woman will need 15mg. We need phosphorus which is used in the chemical reactions that turn food into energy. We need minute quantities, called "trace elements" of copper, cobalt, zinc, manganese, iodine, fluorine and salts. These are found in any diet that includes meat, vegetables, fish and dairy products.

Vitamins are substances required in very small quantities too. Their absence from our diet can lead to deficiency diseases. We need 5000 international units of Vitamin A to keep the skin and the breathing passages healthy. Vitamin B is not a simple vitamin, but a group. B_1 is found in Brewer's Yeast, wheat germ, peas, haricot beans, egg yolk and wholemeal flour. Men need from 1 to 5mg per day, women from 1 to 2mg. B_2 consists of substances usually known by their chemical names. Riboflavin feeds the body cells. Men need 1 to 6mg per day, women 1 to 4mg. It is found in yeast, milk, fish, eggs, and liver. Nicotinic acid helps prevent pellagra and tuberculosis. A man needs 15mg per day, a woman 12mg, and it is found in yeast, liver, fish, meat and wholemeal flour. Folic acid and Vitamin B_{12} help the formation of the blood, and whilst the exact quantities required are not known, folic acid is found in liver and green vegetables, and Vitamin B_{12} in liver, yeast, cereals and pulses. Vitamin C builds healthy tissue. Men need 75mg per day, woman 70mg, and the best sources are fresh fruit, green vegetables, blackcurrants, oranges, lemons, strawberries, apples and cabbage. Vitamin D aids the digestion of calcium. Men and women both need 400 to 800 iu per day. It is found in fish, cod liver oil, halibut liver oil, and in sunlight falling on the skin. Vitamin E is needed for the reproductive system. The exact quantity needed is unknown, but it is found in wheat germ, rice germ, oils, cottonseed oil, lettuce, spinach and eggs. Vitamin K is needed to make the blood clot. It is found in spinach, spring greens, and in dark green vegetables. Vitamin P, called "citrin" makes the capillaries strong. It is found in blackcurrants, oranges, lemons, rose-hips, and green vegetables. Very minute quantities of Vitamins K and P are needed.

Roughage is the name given to indigestible fibres. They simply pass through our bodies, but they help elimination. Constipation arises from the lack of this roughage in our diet, and if persistant, it can lead to colorectal cancer, appendicitis or diverticulitis. Roughage is found in leafy and root vegetables, in fruit, in cereals, in bran and in spinach, but cooking tends to soften these fibres and to make them less effective, so some items should be eaten raw every day.

The other elements we require are fresh air and water. It is vital to give our bodies as much fresh air as possible, sleeping with our window open if we can, and going out into the open air as much as we are able. We must remember, too, that we breathe through our pores as well as our nose, so exposure of the whole body to the air for at least some time during each day is desirable.

Our bodies are composed of between 55 and 70% water. We require an intake of 4 pints (2¼ litres) per day, and we should try to get it from the purest possible source, though bearing in mind that many of our foods already contain water and that this will give us part of our requirement.

Knowing what our daily needs are, it should not be difficult to arrange suitable menus to supply those needs. There are such excellent books on diet that it would be pointless to give another programme here. Remember the desirability of raw natural foods however.

There is an interesting experiment having affinities with dowsing, which you can make with samples of food. It is called the Pendulum Test. Sit facing the magnetic north, with your legs apart. Hold a pendulum, which can be as simple as a button on a thread, in your right hand, so that the pendulum hangs about two inches over a point midway between your knees. You will find after a few moments that it starts to oscillate, swinging away from you and back towards you. Now, take it across so that it hangs over your left knee. After a few moments there, the oscillation will become an ellipse, which will widen gradually into a full circle. Notice whether the pendulum is going around clockwise or anti-clockwise. This varies with the individual, and does not seem to be related to either sex or age. Having found whether you produce a clockwise or an anti-clockwise movement, you are ready to test foods.

Take a sample of the food to be tested in your left hand, and hold it on your palm, using a plate or cup if necessary, midway between your legs. Hold the pendulum in your right hand, so that it is directly over the sample of food under test. Again, the pendulum will begin to oscillate before swinging out into a circle. Note whether the swing is clockwise or anti-clockwise. Those foods which produce the same reaction as you obtained over your left knee are suitable for you; those which produce a swing in the opposite direction are unsuitable. Those which simply produce an oscillation that does not develop into a circle either way are neutral. In doing this test, you must always use your own individual pendulum, never one that someone else has used, and you must bear in mind that impurities in the food or on the dish or cup may produce adverse reactions.

This test may not be foolproof, but it has been known to show up unsuspected allergies, which can then be confirmed in other ways. It would be interesting to see if it confirmed any allergies you know you are suffering from, or how it compared with the foods of which you are particularly fond.

EXERCISE

Exercise is the second way in which we can help ourselves to achieve and maintain fitness. Movement is life. We must be sensible, however, and take into account how much exercise we get in our normal occupation. In the case of a manual worker, this may well be enough, and what he would require in his spare time would be some mental pursuit. Sedentary workers, on the other hand, will certainly need some physical activity.

Probably the best exercise is some sport that we enjoy, because then we shall not look upon it as a task but as a pleasure. There are sports suitable for all ages, and if possible we should choose one that will exercise all our muscle groups. For those of us without heart problems, training with light weights or with chest expanders at home will ensure a balanced routine, if we follow the charts that come with such apparatus.

Walking is an excellent exercise for older people, and has the extra bonus in that it gets them out of the house into the open air. Four miles a day should be adequate to keep fit.

AVOIDANCE OF STRESS

We have already said a lot about stress in the chapter on Meditation. The two killer diseases in Western society today are cancer and coronary thrombosis. Stress helps to bring on one, poor diet the other. It is worthwhile to consider, therefore, what are the causes of stress in our individual lives, and whether we can do anything about them.

Are we in work that fully uses our talents and yet is not beyond our capabilities? Under-employment of our talents can be as frustrating as overloading us with responsibilities we cannot cope with. Do we have a right balance of work and leisure in our lives? Ambition is very good, but to pursue it at the cost of every other enjoyment is not good for our health. Are our personal relationships with family, friends or colleagues all they should be? Does our sex life give to us and to our partner the satisfaction that it should? Are our working conditions poor, noisy or ill-lit? Do fellow workers or supervisors annoy us, or alternatively, if we are supervising, do those under us fail to meet our expectations of them?

All these things can be a cause of stress, and it is best to face them honestly, and to bring our frustrations into the open. People who have a good row and then forget it are doing their health more good than those who bottle up their feelings.

Often we feel that many of the things mentioned above are too personal to discuss with others. We might hesitate to tell the family doctor about them, even if he had time to listen, yet they are relevant to our total health. But trained counsellors, priests, marriage guidance experts, or trustworthy friends make good listeners, and just to express our frustrations and to bring them out into the open can be tremendously helpful. In modern society, the psychiatrist has tended to replace the Father Confessor, but the relief experienced by patient and penitent is essentially the same.

If our self-examination has brought any causes of stress to light, let us consider what we can do about them. It is possible to change jobs, even in these days of high unemployment. We can make more leisure and fill it more happily, if we will accept a different living standard. We can improve our personal relationships, our sex lives, or our working conditions by a different attitude. It is we who allow other people to annoy us. Often the trivialities that upset us are not worth a second's thought, let alone an hour's anger, or a day's brooding, or a lost night's sleep. Anger hurts us far more than the person at whom it is directed. The injunction in The Bible "Let not the sun go down upon your wrath" is good advice from the health point of view as well as the religious.

WATCHING YOUR WEIGHT

The fourth way to help ourselves is to watch our weight. Being overweight makes us susceptible to coronary and renal troubles, to cirrhosis of the liver, to gallstones, and to diabetes mellitus, to mention only a few troubles. Overweight people move more slowly so they do not burn up as many calories as a quick-moving person. Their metabolic rate also slows down, and the whole process becomes a vicious circle.

There are two kinds of excess weight: endogenous and exogenous. Endogenous obesity arises from the improper functioning of one or more of the glands, such as the thyroid, the pituitary, the ovaries or testicles, or the suprarenal glands. This kind of obesity needs medical attention. Exogenous obesity arises from over-eating with too little exercise to burn off the excess. In this we can help ourselves.

There are half a dozen or more diets to help you: the F-Plan, the Scarsdale Diet, the Body Clock Diet, the Mayo Clinic Diet, Weight Watchers, Silhouette. They are all effective if you follow them. All that you need is self-discipline. This is probably where joining one of the Clubs such as Weight Watchers will help you. To be effective, however, a diet must not only enable you to lose weight, it must enable you to stay at your ideal weight. Too many people make a determined effort to reduce weight, only to relax and put all the pounds back on again. You must level out on a diet that you can live with for the rest of your life.

Weight control is simply a matter of balancing the number of calories we put into our bodies with the number we use up. Count the calories you are eating, and try reducing them to 1500 per day, or even 1000 per day for a limited period of not more than two weeks. Weigh before and after this experiment, and see what happens. Weigh once a week, at the same time, preferably first thing in the morning, and stripped. Keep a record. Ignore day to day variations; the weekly check is the true guide. You will soon learn the number of calories you have to reduce to, in order to lose weight, and the number at which you can level out, without putting weight on again. That number must be your diet, and the only way you can increase it is by increasing the amount of physical activities that burn up the extra calories.

PRACTISING RELAXATION

Relaxation is the other way to help yourself keep fit. We have looked at specific techniques of relaxation in the chapter on Meditation. Here we would speak of it in more general terms. Take up some hobby, go to the theatre or concerts, join a sports club, or simply lounge around and do nothing, if that is what you feel like doing. Life should not be one endless rush. There should be time to "stand and stare" as W.H. Davies puts it. Those who make such time are wiser and healthier people.

If, having done all the things suggested in this chapter, you succumb to minor ailments, consider the forms of alternative medicine which you can practise on yourself. Acupressure, Aroma Therapy, the Bach Flower Remedies, Herbalism, Meditation, Shiatzu all offer some scope for self-treatment.

If you rush to the doctor, he may put you on drugs that will have side effects, and simple herbal remedies which you could prepare yourself might be just as effective. A change of diet may be all you need. For example, constipation will respond to spoonfuls of bran in the morning as well as to harsh purgatives. Do not be afraid to experiment. It is your body, and you are the person who will give it the best care.

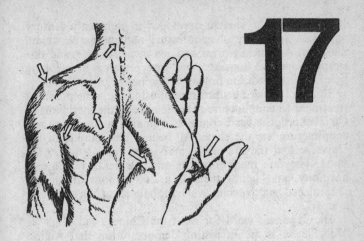

SHIATZU

Shiatzu is the Japanese form of Chinese acupressure. Shi means finger and Atzu pressure. However, whereas the Chinese acupressure uses only the fingers and thumbs, the Japanese Shiatzu uses other parts of the body as well. Sometimes the ball of the thumb, the palm, the elbows, the knees or even the sole of the feet will be used. One technique involves the patient lying on his face whilst the practitioner stands on the soles of his feet. This particular treatment is not as unpleasant as it sounds, and it stimulates the kidneys.

Acupuncture was introduced to Japan from China 1300 years ago. The Japanese have always been adept at taking ideas from other nations, and mixing them with some of their own native cultures to form an amalgam that meets their needs. Thus Japanese judo developed from Chinese martial arts, and Japanese karate from Okinawan methods

In the same way, shiatzu developed in eighteenth century Japan as a mixture of acupressure and the native amma massage. Am means press and ma means stroke, and this simple Japanese massage was just pressing or stroking painful parts with the fingers or the palms of the hands.

Shiatzu followed acupressure in using the same points of treatment as acupuncture. These lie along the meridians of Ch'i. Indeed, the basic concepts of shiatzu, acupressure and acupuncture are the same. All believe that the life of the Universe and the life of the individual are essentially the same. They are made from the same elements, they are in harmony, and hence there is a unity about all things. Diminished health occurs when the balance of Yin and Yang is upset.

The Japanese word for what the Chinese call "Ch'i" is "Ki". There is an interesting demonstration that Aikido masters do, which demonstrates not only the existence of Ki but also its power. Resting their wrist on a partner's shoulder, with the elbow downwards, they will ask the partner to bend their arm by pressing down steadily on the elbow with both hands. Now, if they try to resist this by trying to keep their arm straight, the partner will in most cases succeed in bending it. Try it for yourself; unless the man trying to keep his arm straight is much stronger than the one trying to bend it, the arm will bend at the elbow joint. But now, the Aikido master will show that if, instead of trying to hold his arm rigid, he thinks of it as a fireman's hose, quite limp until filled with water, and then visualizes the power of Ki as being like that water, rushing down his arm and flowing out through his fingers to the whole world, no amount of pressure will make his arm bend. With a little practice anyone can do this. The arm bends at the moment when you lose faith and think "This is not going to work. I have got to try to keep my arm stiff".

Shiatzu became recognised as a therapy in Japan about fifty years ago, when it was codified by Tokojiro Namikoshi. There are now over 20,000 licensed shiatzu therapists in Japan, though it is not as well known in the rest of the world as acupuncture. This is perhaps a pity, since it is free from the risks of infection from dirty needles that might exist with some who call themselves acupuncturists. Moreover the technique is painless.

We know that in ordinary life, touch serves as a means of communication, and just putting our hand on a painful spot can relieve the pain. Lovers hold hands. If we are hurt, we instinctively reach out to the area of pain. Shiatzu scientifically harnesses this principle. Although treatment is given through the fingers or the other points of contact, these are seen only as the outlets for energy. The treatment is truly given with the entire body and with the spirit.

Shiatzu is used for diagnosis and for the prevention of illness as well as for treatment. Some patients have regular sessions in order to avoid becoming ill.

As in all the other alternative therapies, the practitioner will spend a great deal of time at the first session in learning all about his patient. This will be done whether he is being consulted for a particular condition or for general health problems or simply for preventative purposes. The patient's medical history, marital status, work, hobbies, diet are all just as important as to an acupuncturist. Even when he has learned all these facts, the therapist will still rely largely on pulse diagnosis.

Patients are often treated at home, but if they go to a practitioner, they are advised to wear loose-fitting clothing. This not only helps the practitioner; it is more comfortable for the patient. The patient is asked to lie on a couch or even on the floor, while the twelve pulses are being taken. This taking of the pulses is often repeated after treatment as well as before, to assess how the flow of Ki has been affected. The treatment itself can be compared to massage, but it is a very specialised massage, of course, working on the meridians of Ch'i. In Japanese thought, the hara, or stomach, is considered to be the centre of life. It is here that the soul resides, so that in the ritual form of suicide known as seppukku, it is here that the knife is used. Many of the shiatzu treatment points are therefore found in this part of the body.

Pressure is usually applied for a few seconds at a time, and repeated three or four times. This is because, whereas the acupuncturist leaves his needles in and twirls them, the shiatzu therapist is simply pressing on the spot. The fact that such treatment is milder in application is made up for by the repetition. Where the pressure has to be firm enough to cause a certain amount of pain, patients often think of it as pleasurable pain rather than something excruciating, and they rarely complain as they know it is doing them good.

Conditions that respond to shiatzu are those that require pain relief. Headaches, backaches, toothache, depression, constipation and insomnia. Shiatzu is usually used to treat comparatively mild everyday ailments. More serious cases are generally referred to either an acupuncturist or one of the other therapies.

It is not uncommon for patients to practise shiatzu on themselves or even on other members of their family, once they have been shown what to do.

FULL TREATMENT

The full treatment is used to maintain health, and is carried out three or four times a week. It takes about twenty minutes, and can be done to oneself, or by partners to each other. There are sixteen major points of massage:

At the top of each shoulder
At the tip of each shoulder blade
At the outside of the shoulder blades
In the armpits
In the valleys of the thumbs
Above the buttocks
On the points of the elbows
Inside the knees.

A complete treatment like this, when done by a trained therapist, begins at the base of the skull, goes on to the neck muscles, the top of the head, the shoulders, the back, the eyes, the temples, the mouth, under the chin, the neck, the throat, the legs and feet, the hands and arms, and ends up with the patient lying flat on the floor and relaxing. Even the less complicated self-treatment will leave the patient with a sense of inner peace and calm; the full treatment leaves him serene but at the same time full of energy. The shiatzu expert uses no less than six hundred and fifty-seven treatment points.

SPECIAL TREATMENTS FOR SPECIFIC CONDITIONS

(i) For Insomnia

Those who suffer from insomnia have tense neck muscles, so concentration must be given to the neck, shoulders and abdomen. Treatment begins at the top of the head, the base of the skull, the neck muscles, the shoulders, the upper and lower back, the soles of the feet, the abdomen, the front and sides of the neck, and comes back to the temples, the palms of the hands, and the eyes. A session will end with relaxation.

(ii) For Headaches

Headaches are usually caused by fatigue, tension, or over-indulgence in food or alcohol. They can usually be treated in a single session. The head and upper neck muscles will be found to be tense, so the head and shoulders are treated first, going on to the soles of the feet, to improve circulation and to relax the patient.

(iii) For Stiff Neck

This condition is again caused by fatigue or nervous tension. Treatment is first given to the head and neck to open pathways between the head and the heart. The tops of the shoulders, the upper back and the shoulder blades come next. Then the sides and front of the neck, the armpits, the upper arms, and back to the shoulders.

(iv) For Low Back Pain

This is only given where the cause is stress or strain, and must not be given for slipped discs or organic disorders. Treatment is given mainly to the spine and abdomen.

(v) For Constipation or Diarrhoea

Both these may be caused by tension or emotional stress. If the patient is suffering from some abdominal complaint that is responsible for the condition, then shiatzu must not be given.

Where shiatzu is appropriate, it will relax the digestive and intestinal tracts, and so restore normal functioning. Treatment begins at the head and neck to minimise tension and to relax the brain, then goes on to the lower back, and the abdomen to relax the tight muscles there.

Before thinking of self-treatment, consult a trained therapist, who will advise you how to proceed, and even then go back to him if your condition is anything but mild.

A list of qualified shiatzu practitioners can be obtained from The Shiatzu Society (for the address see the Appendix page 152).

CONCLUSION

Readers who look further into the alternatives to orthodox medicine will discover that there are many other therapies besides those dealt with in this book. Indeed, it would be impossible to cover all the existing ones in one volume, and new therapies are being discovered all the time, as the search for alternative healing goes on. Some that you will meet with are full treatments that take care of any condition, others are aids to other forms of treatment rather than complete in their own right. All that can be done in this chapter is to indicate those you are most likely to meet and to offer a guide to where further information can be obtained.

1. ROLFING
This is a manipulative treatment discovered by Ida Rolf, and aims to get the body to take up its natural posture. Apply to the Rolf Institute (for the address see the Appendix page 152).

2. THE ALEXANDER TECHNIQUE
In this, the patient is taught to improve his posture by a trained teacher of the principles. Apply to The Society of Teachers of the Alexander Technique (for the address see the Appendix page 152).

3. THE FELDENKRAIS TECHNIQUE
This again is concerned with posture. The patient unlearns bad postural habits through the medium of movement under the guidance of a teacher. Apply to The Feldenkrais Guild (for the address see the Appendix page 152).

4. YOGA
Yoga concentrates on breathing, posture, and meditation,

and uses exercises. There are many local classes. Apply to The British Wheel of Yoga (for the address see the Appendix page 152).

5. TAI CHI
The exercises in this are based on martial arts movements rather like Kung Fu, but it is a ritual sequence of flowing movement, and is often used to help convalescence. Apply to the British Tai Chi Chuan Association (for the address see the Appendix page 153).

6. DANCE THERAPY
This encourages self-expression through rhythmic movement and is relaxing. Apply to the Natural Dance Association (for the address see the Appendix page 153).

7. ART THERAPY
This encourages self-expression, leading to increased self-knowledge. Apply to the British Association of Art Therapists (for the address see the Appendix page 153).

8. MUSIC THERAPY
Patients may just listen to music, or they may be taught to express themselves through music. Some find this easier than in words. Apply to the Association of Professional Music Therapists (for the address see the Appendix page 153).

9. EXULTATION OF FLOWERS THERAPY
This was discovered by Mr. Alick McInnes, and transfers the healing powers found in plants to water, which is used to raise the body's vital forces in the fight against illness. It has affinities with the Bach Flower Remedies, but Mr. McInnes's book is out of print and difficult to obtain.

10. IONISATION
The theory behind this is that men and women function better when the negative particles in the air are increased. Machines can be bought which do this, both in the home and in factories, where they are said to lead to significant

improvement in work performance.

11. THE METAMORPHIC TECHNIQUE
This uses reflex points rather like reflexology. The country's leading practitioner is Gaston Saint-Pierre. Apply to the Metamorphic Association (for the address see the Appendix page 153).

In all the therapies we have been considering in this book, there are certain common factors:

(i) They all believe in the power of the body to right itself, given favourable conditions.
(ii) The theme of "harmony" runs through many of them. It is found in acupuncture, acupressure, the Bach Flower Remedies, healing, mantra, shiatzu, and others. The Universe is conceived as being harmonious.
(iii) All agree that man is more than just his physical body, and that healing cannot be on the physical plane alone.
(iv) Many believe in a benevolent power in the Universe, that Christians would call "God".

These common factors link the therapies with the great religions of the world, and give a spiritual dimension to healing.

It would be wrong if anything in this book disparaged the very real achievements of orthodox medicine. Doctors are in the healing profession just as much as alternative practitioners, and their successes are many. But in cases where the best efforts of medical science are not enough, or their methods are rejected for any of the reasons given in the Introduction, it is worth remembering that there is not just one other way. There are many.

APPENDIX

For addresses of acupuncturists write to:

The British Acupuncture Association and Register, 34 Alderney Street, London, SW1V 4EV.
(Members of this register will have had either medical or naturopathic training in addition to acupuncture, and after a two or three year course will hold the qualifications M.B.Ac.A. or F.B.Ac.A.)

The College of Traditional Chinese Acupuncture, Queensway, Leamington Spa, Warwickshire.
(Students of this college take a two or three year course and hold the qualifications Lic.Ac. or B.Ac.)

The International College of Oriental Medicine, Green Hedges Avenue, East Grinstead, Sussex, RH19 1DZ.
(Students take a two or three year course and qualify as B.Ac. or D.Ac.)

For addresses of aromatherapists write to:

The Secretary, NDA, 42A Hillfield Park, London, N10.

The Wealden Natural Health Clinic, 1 Clanricade Gardens, Tunbridge Wells, Kent.

The College of Natural Therapies, 22 Bromley Road, London SE6.

Suppliers of oils for Aroma Therapy:

Hartwood Aromatics, 12 Station Road, Hatton, Warwick, OU35 7LG.

Celeste Aromatics, 26 Foxbourne Road, London SW17.

To obtain Dr. Bach's flower remedies write to:

The Dr. Edward Bach Centre, Mount Vernon, Sotwell, Wallingford, Oxon, OX10 OPZ.
(Dr. Bach's books published by C. W. Daniel Co. are available from the centre.)

Chiropractic

Anglo-European College of Chiropractic, 2 Cavendish Road, Bournemouth, Dorset, BH1 1RA.

The British Chiropractor's Association, 5 First Avenue, Chelmsford, Essex, CM1 1RX.

Health Clinics, Health Farms and Spas:

Inglewood Health Hydro, Templeton Road, Kingbury, Berkshire.

Tyringham Clinic, near Newport Pagnall, Buckinghamshire.

Champneys, Tring Health Resort, Tring, Hertfordshire.

Champneys, Stobo Health & Beauty Resort, Stobo, Peebles, Scotland.

For those suffering from cancer:

The Cancer Help Centre, 7 Downfield Road, Clifton, Bristol, BS8 2TG.

The Association for New Approaches to Cancer (A.N.A.C.), 28 Blythe Road, London, W14 0HA.

For addresses of spiritualists write to:

The Churches Council for Health & Healing, Marylebone Road, London, NW1 5LT.

Fountain Trust, 3A High Street, Esher, Surrey, KT10 9RP.

National Federation of Spiritualist Healers, Church Street, Sunbury-on-Thames, Middlesex, TW16 6RG.

The Harry Edwards Spiritual Sanctuary, Burrows Lane, Shere, Guildford, Surrey.

For addresses of homoeopaths write to:

The Faculty of Homoeopathy, Royal London Homoeopathic Hospital, Great Ormond Street, London, WC1.

The Society of Homoeopaths, 59 Norfolk House Road, London, SW12.

The British Homoeopathic Association, 27A Devonshire Street, London, W1N 1RJ.

The Hahnemann Society, Humane Education Centre, Avenue Lodge, Bounds Green Road, London, N22 4EV.

The Society of Homoeopaths, 101 Sebastian Avenue, Shenfield, Brentwood, Essex, CM15 8PP.

The Unani system of herbal medicine

The Association of Unani and Ayurvedic Practitioners, 12 Little Newport Street, London, W1.

Herbal medicine

The National Institute of Medical Herbalists, 41 Hatherley Road, Winchester, Hants, SO22 6RR.

Naturopathy

The British Naturopathic & Osteopathic Association, 6 Netherhall Gardens, London, NW3 5RR.

Iridiology

The School of Iridiology & Wholistic Healing, Bright Haven, Robins Lane, Lolworth, Cambridge, CB3 8HH.

Colleges of Osteopathy

The British School of Osteopathy, 1–4 Suffolk Street, London, SW1Y 4HG.

The British College of Osteopathy & Naturopathy, 6 Netherhall Gardens, London, NW3 5RR.

The European School of Osteopathy, 104 Tonbridge Road, Maidstone, Kent.

Radionics

The Radionic Association, 16A North Bar, Banbury, Oxon.

Reflexology

The Bayley School of Reflexology, Monks Orchard, Whitbourne, Worcester, WR6 5RB.

International Institute of Reflexology, P O Box 34, Harlow, Essex, CM17 0LT.

The Crusade Against All Cruelty to Animals Ltd., Humane Education Centre, Avenue Lodge, Bounds Green Road, London, N22 4EV.

Shiatzu

The Shiatzu Society, 11 Ivydene Road, Reading, RG3 1HT.

Rolfing

Rolf Institute, P O Box 1868, Boulder, Colorado, 80302, U.S.A.

The Alexander Technique

The Society of Teachers of the Alexander Technique, 36 Albert Court, Kensington Gore, London, SW7.

The Feldenkrais Technique

Feldenkrais Guild, 4 The Broadway, Wimbledon, London, SW19.

Yoga

The British Wheel of Yoga, 80 Lechampton Road, Cheltenham, Gloucester.

Tai Chi

British Tai Chi Chuan Association, 7 Upper Wimpole Street, London, W1M 7TD.

Dance Therapy

Natural Dance Association, 14 Peto Place, London, NW1 4DT.

Art Therapy

British Association of Art Therapists, 13C Northwood Road, London, N6 5LT.

Music Therapy

Association of Professional Music Therapists, 22 Ermine Street, Caxton, Cambs., CB3 8PQ.

The Metamorphic Technique

Metamorphic Association, 67 Ritherdon Road, London, SW17 8QE.

Source of Products

Some of the products mentioned in this book can be obtained from branches of "The Body Shop", of which there are over 60 in the U.K., with many more overseas. Information on this organisation can be had by sending a stamped self-addressed envelope to: The Body Shop International plc, Dominion Way, Rustington, West Sussex BN16 3LR, U.K.

INDEX

OUR PUBLISHING POLICY

HOW WE CHOOSE

0800606900

Our policy is to consider every deserving manuscript and we can give special editorial help where an author is an authority on his subject but an inexperienced writer. We are rigorously selective in the choice of books we publish. We set the highest standards of editorial quality and accuracy. This means that a *Paperfront* is easy to understand and delightful to read. Where illustrations are necessary to convey points of detail, these are drawn up by a subject specialist artist from our panel.

HOW WE KEEP PRICES LOW

We aim for the big seller. This enables us to order enormous print runs and achieve the lowest price for you. Unfortunately, this means that you will not find in the *Paperfront* list any titles on obscure subjects of minority interest only. These could not be printed in large enough quantities to be sold for the low price at which we offer this series.
We sell almost all our *Paperfronts* at the same unit price. This saves a lot of fiddling about in our clerical departments and helps us to give you world-beating value. Under this system, the longer titles are offered at a price which we believe to be unmatched by any publisher in the world.

OUR DISTRIBUTION SYSTEM

Because of the competitive price, and the rapid turnover, *Paperfronts* are possibly the most profitable line a bookseller can handle. They are stocked by the best bookshops all over the world. It may be that your bookseller has run out of stock of a particular title. If so, he can order more from us at any time—we have a fine reputation for "same day" despatch, and we supply any order, however small (even a single copy), to any bookseller who has an account with us. We prefer you to buy from your bookseller, as this reminds him of the strong underlying public demand for *Paperfronts*. Members of the public who live in remote places, or who are housebound, or whose local bookseller is unco-operative, can order direct from us by post.

FREE

If you would like an up-to-date list of all paperfront titles currently available, send a stamped self-addressed envelope to
ELLIOT RIGHT WAY BOOKS, BRIGHTON RD.,
LOWER KINGSWOOD, SURREY, U.K.